CW00815730

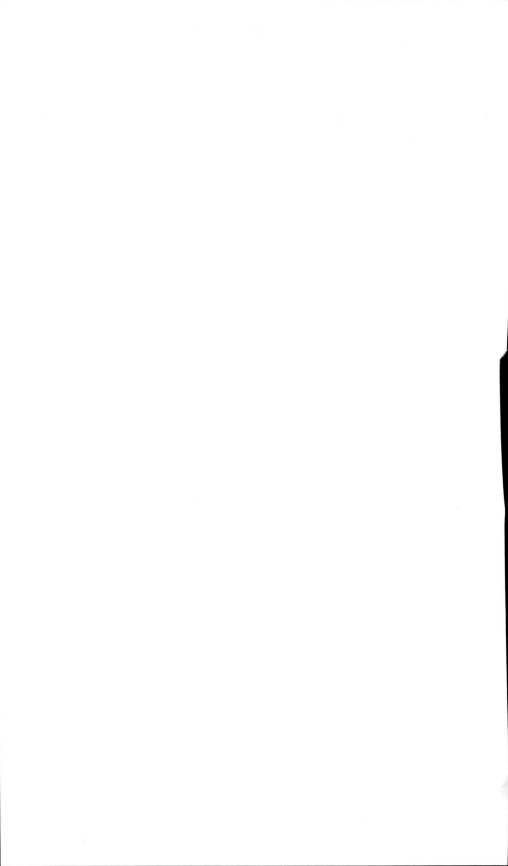

Dash Diet for Beginners

The Perfect Action Plan with a 28-Day Weight Loss Program and a Meal Plan Solution to Lower Hypertension and Blood Pressure, Prevent Diabetes and Improve Your Health

Maria Crawford

Table of Contents

Introduction

Congratulations on downloading the *Dash Diet for Beginners*. This eBook aims to give you information about the dash diet and how you can implement it in your life. Thank you for taking the time to download this book.

The author of this book has carried out a lot of research to compile the information on this book. This is not the only information there is pertaining to the diet. However, the information here is deemed to be true. Some of the information here is already available online but has been placed in this book for your easy retrieval.

Finally, a big thanks to you the reader for choosing to read this book! There are a lot of books online which are similar to this one, but out of all of them, you choose to read this one. Thank you!

Chapter 1: Dash Diet: How it Works and its Benefits

DASH Diet Explained

DASH is an abbreviation for Dietary Approaches to Stop Hypertension. It is recommended as a remedy for those suffering from hypertension and a preventive measure for those with normal blood pressure.

DASH recommends a dietary lifestyle change as opposed to quick fixes. You are encouraged to eat a wide range of nutrient-dense foods mainly fruits, low-fat dairy products, lean meats, vegetables, and whole grains. Another essential component of the diet is reduced sodium intake.

Sodium and Hypertension

What has sodium got to do with blood pressure? Well, a lot. Let us start with the kidneys, which are tasked with the essential role of removing extra fluids from the body after filtering the blood. The extra fluid is directed to the bladder and eliminated from the body as urine. This process uses osmosis, which requires a delicate balance of potassium and sodium.

Eating excess sodium, which is basically salt in your diet, ruins this balance compromising the effectiveness of your kidneys in eliminating the fluids.

You may have noticed that when you eat salty food, you pee less frequently. In fact, before a long journey or when going to a function where the bathroom is not readily accessible, some people will eat a pinch of salt and this will effectively keep their bladder from filling for hours.

While such one-off instances maybe harmless, a constant intake of sodium raises blood pressure due to the excess fluid. The strain put on the kidney can lead to kidney disease, which will in turn cause toxins to accumulate in the body. The arteries are affected as well. The extra blood pressure caused by the excess fluid strains the arteries and the tiny muscles in their walls become thicker while attempting to keep up with the pumping. Thicker muscles mean that the space inside the arteries is reduced, raising the blood pressure even higher as it is now being forced through a constricted space.

For these reasons, there is a specific version of the DASH diet that pays precise attention to the amount of salt in the diet, recommending a maximum of 2,300 mg of sodium a day. If you're already suffering from hypertension, your daily limit should not exceed 1,500mg. Note that the American's average diet is consists of up to 3,400mg of sodium in a single day.

Even when you do not add a single grain of salt to your food, there's already so much of it in processed foods. This is one of the reasons why the DASH diet highly recommends fresh foods.

You can reduce your sodium intake by getting a substitute for table salt in your food. There are several natural spices such as ginger or garlic that have that sour tinge that you crave for in salt. Another alternative is to sprinkle fresh lemon juice, especially on meat.

Rinse canned foods before cooking. Most of them come soaked with a salty sauce which you can do away with. How about processed meat? Check the labels for sodium content. Sausages, hot dogs, bacon, ham, and the like tend to be extra salty. If you cannot find a sodium-free/low option, which is mostly the case, stay away from them altogether. Finally, remove that salt shaker from the dinner table. Sometimes the act of adding salt is purely psychological, with some people adding even before they taste the food. Even in a restaurant, ask the waiter to take it back. Once it's out of sight, chances are, you won't even need it.

History of the DASH diet

DASH diet dates back to the early 1990s when concern was raised about the prevalence of lifestyle diseases, among them hypertension. In 1992, under the funding of the National

Institute of Health (NIH), several research projects were initiated to determine if dietary changes could be effective in treating hypertension.

The participants were provided with a meal plan and advised not to include any other lifestyle modification so that all the changes could be attributed directly to the dietary interventions.

The results were encouraging. A decrease of about 6 to 11 mm Hg was reported in systolic blood pressure in a span of a few weeks. In addition, the lower levels of sodium in the diet dropped, the lower the blood pressure dropped. In addition to reducing hypertension, the cholesterol levels were reduced as well.

After several subsequent studies and experiments with positive results, the DASH diet became and still is highly recommended as a long-term remedy for hypertension.

Foods in the DASH Diet

The DASH diet allows a variety of foods rich in nutrients such as calcium, potassium, and magnesium. The food groups involved include legumes, nuts, lean meats, low-fat dairy products, whole grains, fruits, vegetables, and some fats. These ingredients are low in cholesterol and saturated fats, limiting the daily calorie intake to a healthy 2,000 on average.

Here are some ideas on how to incorporate these food groups in your diet:

1. Whole Grains

Most of the grains in the market today are processed, making them more sugary and most people will opt for this category. Whole grains might be less appealing to your taste-buds, but your body will eventually thank you. The outer brown coat that is removed during processing is rich in nutrients and most importantly, fiber. Go for whole-wheat pasta, whole grain bread, brown rice, whole grain cereal, and so on. Even when selecting flour for your own baking, go for the unprocessed option. Be sure to read the labels before purchasing. Some brands have been known to add a brown color so the products appear as whole grains while they're really not.

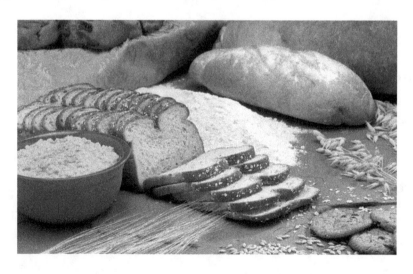

2. Nuts/Legumes

They include peanuts, lentils, kidney beans, almonds, soybeans, and so on. They provide rich sources of potassium, magnesium, and proteins. Different colors of legumes/grains represent certain nutrients. You will find that they come in a wide range of colors including red, maroon, yellow, cream, white, and so on. Try to incorporate as many of them as possible over time so you can benefit from all the nutrients. Take nuts in moderation; they're high in calories and could jeopardize your daily calorie intake.

Another major advantage of nuts and legumes is their filling ability. Incorporating them into your meal leaves you feeling fuller for longer. This way, you're less likely to snack on unhealthy options. You can also substitute meat with them as a source of protein.

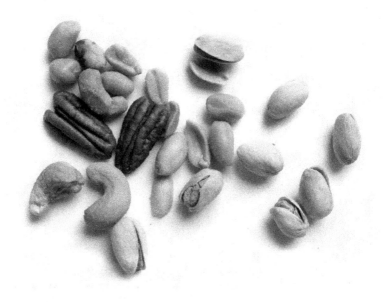

3. Vegetables

The vegetable song is not going away any time soon. From when you were a kid and were forced to eat your vegetables, to an adult still having to deal with the same notion. Why are vegetables deemed unpleasant again? Well, let's admit that most of them are not exactly tasty. We prefer something that is more tantalizing to our taste buds.

Vegetables do not have to be boring though. Carrots, kales, cabbage, beetroot, broccoli, name them. With all their different colors and textures, you can sure turn them into something palatable. Experiment with different combinations and different styles of cooking. For all the vitamins, minerals, and fiber that they give you, they're definitely worth the effort. Do not think of vegetables as a side thing. Let them be part of the main course. In fact, aim for half of your plate to consist of vegetables.

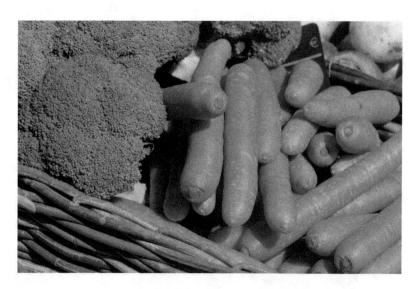

4. Fruits

Rich in fiber and vitamins and come in several great flavors. Whether you prefer one fruit at a time or you mix them into a salad, you can enjoy them either with your meal or as a snack. Talking of snacks, fruits provide a great snacking option so you don't have to go for sugary or fatty fast foods. Always pack a few fruits with you so you have something to bite on whenever you're hungry.

Is fruit juice a substitute for fruits? Well, although the juice contains similar nutrients, it takes away the fiber which is essential for digestion. Is it advisable to eat the fruits themselves whenever you can? For those with edible peels such as apples, pears, and plums, eat the peels; they have their own extra set of nutrients.

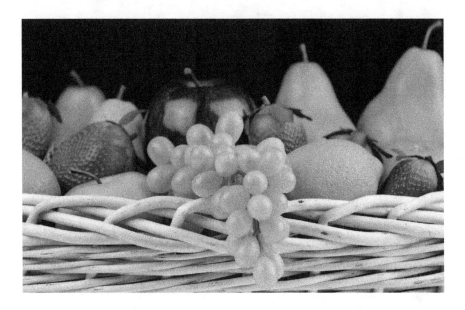

5. Lean Meats

The DASH diet does not advocate for doing away with meat entirely, but for eating it with moderation as it remains a rich source of protein, Vitamin B, zinc, and iron. You can have your meat twice a week or so, favoring white meat over red meat. When cooking chicken, remove the skin which holds most of the fat. With red meat, remove the fatty areas. Let the meat occupy only a quarter of your plate, with the rest being shared between vegetables and whole grain carbs.

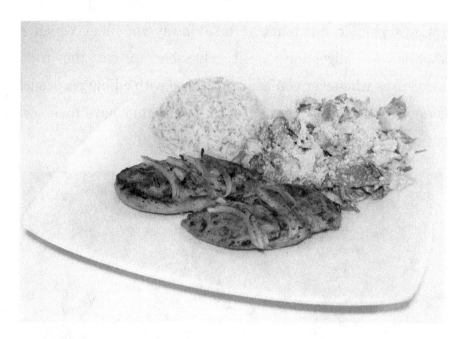

6. Dairy Products

For their Vitamin D and Calcium content, dairy products remain part of the DASH diet. Go for milk, yogurt, and cheese that are labeled low-fat or even fat-free. Dairy products ordinarily contain that saturated type of fat, which is to be avoided at all cost. Chilled yogurt makes a great snack and you can add fruit pieces or nuts to spruce it up. When buying cheese, check for a low-sodium option.

Generally, avoid foods with excess salt, sugar, fat, or processed foods. Even though some of these foods may not affect your blood pressure directly, they increase the chances of other lifestyle diseases like obesity and heart conditions, which in turn cause hypertension.

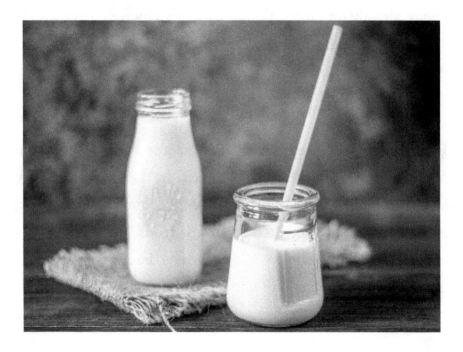

Benefits of the DASH Diet

For a diet that was formulated to treat hypertension and which in most cases has successfully done so, the DASH diet has so many additional benefits. It is basically healthy eating so the body benefits in multiple aspects. Even if you're not suffering from high blood pressure, DASH diet is still highly recommended. It'll go a long way in helping you avoid the condition as well as other lifestyle diseases such as diabetes, obesity, and heart disease.

If you're already suffering from hypertension, this diet can help you ease the symptoms which include headaches, chest pains, fatigue, labored breathing, and irregular heartbeat. Even if you're already on medication, the dietary changes will regulate your blood pressure so you don't have to live on medication. Additional benefits include:

1. More Nutritious Meals

Eliminating processed foods and incorporating more fresh foods gives you healthy meals which are beneficial to every aspect of your being. Adjusting may take some effort at first, especially if you're accustomed to fast foods, but the result is very well worth the effort. You will reduce the chances of health issues throughout your lifetime and enjoy a largely vibrant, pain-free life.

2. Healthier Kidneys

The nutrients found in the DASH eating plan including potassium, calcium, magnesium, and fiber nourish every part of the body and the kidneys are no exception. In addition, the lower consumption of sodium as recommended further favor the kidneys allowing them to filter blood efficiently.

3. Prevent Diabetes

Diabetes is caused largely by insulin resistance. The DASH diet is tried and tested in curbing insulin resistance. If you're already suffering from diabetes, you can be certain of experiencing some relief. For those predisposed to the disease due to genetic factors, this can only prevent or delay the onset of diabetes.

4. Reduced Risk of Heart Disease

High blood pressure strains the heart, as it is required to pump harder to facilitate circulation. With the blood pressure regulated, the heart works comfortably reducing the risk of developing problems. For those already living with heart disease, the diet eases the burden and increases the chances of restoration of normal heart operations.

5. Reduce and Regulate Body Weight

By limiting the calories and saturated fats, this diet will help you shed extra pounds if you're overweight and maintain a healthy body weight once you've achieved it. By shedding excess body weight, which is essentially fat, you reduce the risk of the above health conditions and are able to remain active.

Transitioning to the DASH Diet

As any other life adjustment, it is not easy at the start. Most people associate the idea of dieting with hunger pangs, boring tasteless food, reduced options, and an all-around misery that they just have to endure. Going by the information above, you must have noted that the DASH diet is different. It is not a list of stringent rules and scores of foods that you cannot eat. It is flexible, still allowing you to enjoy a wide array of foods, with moderation. Here are some tips to help you get started on the DASH diet:

Change slowly

You don't have to throw out your current supplies and get a whole new shopping list. Such a drastic change is not good for your body, which needs time to get accustomed to new foods. It is not good for your emotions either, there's a sense of oppression that comes with having foods forced down your throat; literally, in this case. Begin, for instance, by changing your snacks. Instead of a bar of chocolate or a cookie, carry a fruit or some peanuts. Insist on carrying, the healthy options may not be available for purchase when the hunger pangs strike.

Proceed to your plate. Gradually replace the animal proteins with the plant-based ones. Include more vegetables. Go for light vegetable-based cooking oil as opposed to cooking fats. With time, the changes get easier.

Cook at home

Eating out does not give you many healthy options. You may scrutinize the menu to the very last option, but you can't really tell the ingredients in every meal. A vegetarian option may be the closest you'll get to a meal that adheres to the DASH diet.

Why not prepare your own meals at home? No matter how busy you are, you sure can squeeze in an extra hour that will have a positive impact on your health. Start by looking for interesting recipes then shopping for the ingredients. That will get you in the mood for cooking. Cook a lot of food at a time and refrigerate/freeze in portions, so you do not have to cook from scratch each time. Chop the vegetables before refrigerating them, so you can have them ready in minutes when you need them.

Exercise

Diet plans hardly ever work in isolation. Add some physical activity into your routine. Go to the gym, walk, jog, run, cycle, dance, stretch, or do whatever else is at your disposal. Exercise helps reduce body fat, some of which may have been deposited in blood vessels further worsening the hypertension. A diet-exercise combination steadily reduces the blood pressure and maintains it at that healthy level.

Get Company

Join a community of other people following the DASH diet. Here you will trade experiences, share recipes, gauge progress, and generally get adequate support.

For all the benefits it harbors, the DASH diet is well worth the effort. With time, you even forget that you're on a diet, you simply turn healthy eating into a lifestyle. And for that, you increase your chances of lifelong wellness of body and mind.

Chapter 2: What Are the Dietary Approaches Towards Hypertension?

Taking up the DASH diet is a proven way that doctors highly recommend to help lower a person's high blood pressure or prevent their blood pressure from rising. This lowers your risk of developing heart disease, hypertension, and diabetes.

The diet is basically characterized by foods that have lower quantities of sodium. Instead, the foods are rich in other nutrients such as magnesium, calcium, and potassium. These three nutrients can really help to lower the blood pressure. A typical DASH diet is characterized by plenty of fruits, vegetables, and dairy products that have low-fat content. Nuts, whole grains, fish, and poultry are a great component of the diet. Sweets, lean meat, and some sugary beverages are also offered but in limited portions.

Low Sodium Version of the DASH Diet

To limit the intake of foods that increase the sodium levels in the body is the main emphasis of the dash diet. This is the standard DASH diet. However, there are some versions of the diet that have lower sodium levels. These provisions are meant to fit one's health needs. They include:

- The Lower Sodium DASH diet: This version of the diet allows you to take 1,500mg of sodium in a day.

- The Standard DASH diet: This version gives an allowance to consume 2,300mg of sodium in a day.

Sticking to a typical American diet means that you consume about 3,400 milligrams or more sodium in a day. This amount is very high and works against the goal of reducing your blood pressure. The lower sodium and the standard DASH diets allow for the intake of food with sodium but ensure that you adhere to the recommended sodium intake amount to less than 2,300 milligrams in a day.

The lower sodium DASH diet is the most preferred of the two given it assures you of adhering to the set limits. However, it is always advisable to consult with your doctor to know the sodium levels that are right for you.

Recommended Servings for Different Food Groups in the DASH Diet

Given that the diet is rich in whole grains, vegetables, fruits, lean meat, and dairy products with low-fat content, this section aims at giving a general guide of the recommended servings that will help you adhere to the 2000 calories recommended in a day.

Grains Servings

Purpose to have between 6 and 8 serving of grain in a day. This could be cereal, bread, pasta, or rice. An ounce of dry cereal, a single slice of whole-wheat bread, or half a cup of cooked rice, pasta, or cereal amount to one serving.

It is advisable that you focus more on the whole grains. They are richer in nutrients and fiber as compared to refined grains. So when grocery shopping, go for the brown sugar rice, whole-grain bread, and whole-wheat pasta. Always keep an eye on products with the "100% whole grain" label. Also, when preparing your grains, avoid adding cheese, cream, or butter sauces. Naturally, grains have low-fat content. You should try to keep them that way.

Fruits Servings

The beauty of fruits is that they do require little to no time to prepare. And they can be taken as snacks or as part of a whole meal. Fruits, just like vegetables, are very rich in potassium, magnesium, and fiber. They also have low-fat content, with coconuts being the only exception.

The DASH diet recommended fruits servings are between 4 and 5 in a day. A single serving can be one whole fruit or half a cup of frozen or canned fruit. 4 ounces of a pure fruit juice is also equal to one serving.

You should strive to have at least a piece of fruit after every meal and another piece as a snack in between meals. A dessert of fresh fruits after an evening meal is a great way to round out your day. If you are consuming canned fruits or fruit juice, ensure that there is no added sugar in them. For the juice, ensure that it is fresh fruit juice with no chemical additives.

Whenever possible, you should leave and consume edible peels too. Fruits like apples, pears, and even mangoes have edible peels. These peels offer additional nutrient, fiber, and texture to the recipe.

While fruits are generally recommended, you should be cautious with regards to the fruit you are consuming. Some fruits, especially citrus fruits and juices, could have some effect on the medication you are taking. As such, if you are under any medication, consult with your doctor to know whether such fruits are okay to consume.

Vegetable Servings

Just like fruits, it is recommended to have between 4 and 5 vegetable servings in a day. 1 cup of leafy vegetables (raw) or 1/2 cup of cut-up raw or cooked cut-up vegetables amounts to one serving. The most common and most preferred vegetables for the DASH diet include carrots, tomatoes, greens, broccoli, and sweet potatoes. These vegetables are rich in minerals such as magnesium and potassium. They also have very high vitamin and fiber content.

Vegetables are a great choice given they can be added to any meal. They can also be taken as the main dish and not just as a side dish as many people do. Again, when shopping for vegetables, go for the fresh ones. If you are buying canned or frozen vegetables, ensure that they have low sodium content.

Dairy Servings

2 to 3 servings of a dairy product are enough to get you through the day. Milk, cheese, and yogurt are mostly preferred. They are very rich in vitamin D, protein, and calcium. But you ought to be careful when choosing the dairy products to add to your meal. One of the main characteristics of a DASH diet is the low-fat content. Some dairy products have high-fat content. You should avoid such.

A single dairy serving can be comprised of 1 cup of low-fat yogurt, skim, or milk. 1 ½ ounce of part-skim cheese also amounts to a single serving.

Adding frozen yogurt with low or no fat is a great way of boosting the number of dairy products you consume. Yogurt also offers a sweet treat guaranteeing you that you will enjoy your meal.

Go for lactose-free products or an over-the-counter dairy product if you are lactose intolerant. Also, go easy on the cheese. They typically have high sodium levels.

Lean Meat, Fish, and Poultry Servings

If you are like most people, chances are that meat is one of the key components of your meals. Meat is rich in proteins, zinc, iron, and B vitamins. With the DASH diet, the lean meat varieties are the most preferred. It is recommended that you have a maximum of 6 serving or less of lean meat in a day. To make your meal healthier, cut back on the meat and add more vegetables. This would provide a healthier diet as compared to having more of the meat and less of the vegetables.

With meat, fat is always concentrated under the skin. As such, trim away the skin and the fat from the meat before you prepare the meat. Also, instead of frying the meat, grill, roast, or broil it. This ensures that the excess fat is shed off. Frying only means that the meat will soak in more fat, thus increasing the fat content in your meal; something you are trying to reduce on.

Fish like herring, salmon, and tuna have high omega-3 content, helpful in lowering your cholesterol levels.

Seeds, Legumes, and Nuts Servings

The recommended servings for seeds, nuts, and legumes are 4 to 5 in a week. These foods are a good source of protein, potassium, and magnesium. They also come with high fiber and phytochemicals levels helpful in protecting you against cardiovascular disease and some cancers.

The recommended servings are relatively small with the consumption limited to just a few times in a week. The reason for this is that these foods are rich in calories. A single serving is equivalent to 2 tablespoons of seeds, half a cup of cooked peas or bean, or a third cup of nuts.

When consuming nuts, add salads or cereals for a healthier meal. Also, you can use seeds and legumes as an alternative if you do not take meat. Products of Soybeans are particularly great.

Sweets Servings

You can also incorporate sweets in your DASH diet. You only have to be careful to limit your intake of the same. The most servings you can have in a week is 5. A tablespoon of jelly, sugar or jam, 1 cup of lemonade, or ½ cup sorbet is equivalent to one serving.

Again, the rules do not change. Stick to those sweets that are low on fat or those that have no fat at all. Sorbet, jelly beans, graham crackers, fruit ices, or low-fat cookies are great choices to consider. Avoid added sugar at all cost. It offers no nutritional value. You will only be adding to your calories.

Fats and Oils Servings

Fats are helpful in helping your body absorb and utilize essential vitamins. They also are helpful in ensuring your immune system functions effectively. However, when in excess, fats can be quite harmful. The excess of fats increase the chances of you being obese, getting diabetes, or developing heart disease.

The DASH diet ensures that you consume just the right amount of fats to keep your body healthy. 2 to 3 servings per day are recommended. 1 teaspoon of soft margarine, 2 tablespoons of salad dressing, or a tablespoon of mayonnaise amount to one serving.

Also, make sure to limit the consumption of foods that are rich in fats such as meat, cheese, whole milk, eggs, and butter among others. You also should be cautious of trans-fat that is common on fried items, baked good, and other processed foods.

When doing your grocery shopping, always read the labels of the products you are buying. Choose those that are free of trans fat and those that have the lowest saturated fat.

DASH Diet Beverages

There are so many healthy beverage options to choose from these days. You, therefore, shouldn't find it difficult to find a suitable beverage or drink. Here are some healthy options of drinks and beverages to quench your thirst.

1. Water

This is an obvious one. It comes top of the list since it is the healthiest, and perhaps, the most readily available drink. It is recommended that a person consumes 8 glasses of water in a day. Since it can be difficult to attain the recommended number of glasses, you can compensate by consuming foods that have high water content such as fleshy fruits and vegetables. Another option is to make soup using other products such as meat and legumes.

The important thing is to ensure you consume a lot of water daily.

2. Coffee

Another great drink with low calories is coffee. The best coffee is made of espresso and water only. This might sound a bit flat and you might think of making it better by adding some of your favorite ingredients. Don't. Get rid of your sweet tooth. The more the ingredients you add, the more calories you add in the coffee.

The transition to taking plain coffee can be a bit challenging at first. But the more you take it, the more you will get used to it. It also is more beneficial to your health in the long run.

3. Tea

Tea is another great beverage to take if you are on a DASH diet. Tea slows the rate of sugar intake in the body, hence regulating your blood sugar levels.

Hibiscus tea is one of the most effective beverages to take if you are on the DASH diet. This tea contains anthocyanins among antioxidants that help prevent blood vessels from being narrow. It is one of those "fast-action" beverages.

4. Smoothies

You can enjoy a DASH diet smoothie. You can get yourself a turmeric smoothie, a skinny margarita, or a spicy Bloody Mary to accompany your meal.

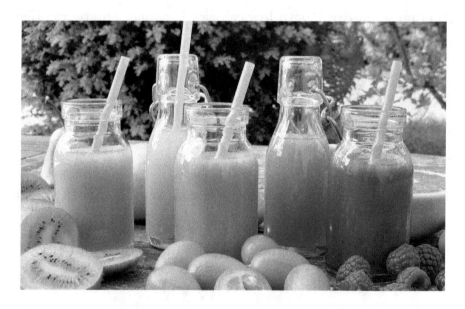

5. Pomegranate Juice

Pomegranate juice has been proven to increase a person's systolic blood pressure. Its antioxidant activity is three times that of green tea. It is a great drink to take if you are on the DASH diet.

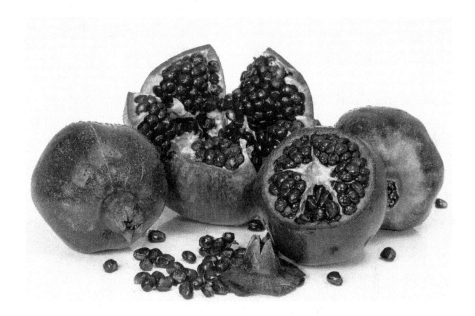

Some Alcohol?

It has been proven that when you drink too much alcohol, chances of your blood pressure increasing shoot up drastically. With this knowledge, if you are on the DASH diet, you should limit your alcohol consumption to the recommended levels. Women should stick to the one drink or less limit in a day. Men's limit is set at two drinks or less in a day.

Staying True to the DASH Diet

If you are used to taking meat every day, cutting back on your consumption as the diet requires can be a bit challenging. Same applies to consuming other products that are your favorite but have high calories. You need to have a strategy to make it work. Here are some tips that will help you transition fully to the DASH diet and help you stay true to it.

Make a gradual change

The trick to changing a habit is by cutting back on some of the things you love slowly. For instance, if you only take vegetables or fruits once in a day, try adding an additional serving either during lunchtime or at dinner. Once you get used to it, add another serving and gradually increase them until you attain the recommended number of servings in a day.

Same applies when cutting back on your consumption. If you are used to having 4 alcohol drinks in a day, try reducing them gradually. Start taking 3 first, then 2, then one.

The gradual change makes it easier for you and your body to adjust to the new system.

Do not be too hard on yourself

This only means that you should always find a reason to reward yourself with every progress that you make. Be careful though. The rewards should always be nonfood. Rewards can be taking yourself out for a movie or even buying yourself a gift. The more you reward yourself, the more motivated you get to adhering to the diet and achieving more.

If you happen to slip, don't be discouraged. Change can be a tough process. In the event that you slip, pick yourself up and continue from where you left off.

Add physical activity into the mix

Engaging in physical activity is one of the great ways to complement your DASH diet. Exercising greatly helps in lowering your blood pressure. A combination of the diet and physical activities helps you achieve your goal much faster.

You don't have to do it alone

Picking up a new habit is difficult. But the good thing is that you do not have to do it alone. If you are having a difficult time transitioning and adhering to the diet, you can find yourself a friend or a loved one to help you by keeping you accountable. You can also always talk to your doctor for help.

DASH diet aims to help you eat healthily and still be able to lower your blood pressure. The foods covered in the diet are plenty, offering you a lot of flexibility with regards to what and what not to include in your meal. The meal plans and menus are plenty. What you should ensure is that the approach you employ is within the recommended limits. That way, you will get to live healthier.

Chapter 3: What Are the Dietary Approaches for Weight Loss via the Dash Diet?

The DASH diet program is among the best program introduced by the health care that has come to help a lot of people with related issues like body size, high and low blood pressure, and hypertension. This program is not only initiated to keep patients disease free but also implemented to keep people fit.

In this blog, you will be learning the best ways of losing weight within a month and how effective the result is. Other than that, you will be learning on various ways to maintaining a proper body size through proper workouts and proper meal plan. At the end of this, be sure that your body will be disease free and very flexible through the best weight loss workouts.

Below are some of the reasons why you definitely need to reduce weight and watch out for obesity or overweight.

- High and low blood pressure
  Blood pressure is among the leading challenges in overweight and the result is very severe. Blood pressure should be keenly watched out for and detected first and necessary actions to be taken. It is known to lead to bad headaches that cause stress, strokes which may lead to

death if taken lightly, or even nose bleeding as the blood pumps in the body with a lot of pressure.

- Pregnancy challenges

Overweight often leads to pregnancy risks especially in obesity cases and the result is that most of the time, the mothers have to go under C-section for deliverance, for the safety of the baby. I wouldn't recommend C-section method as it is always painful and dangerous sometimes.

- Kidney diseases

Overweight most of the time is known to lead to chronic kidney disease which is normally brought by excessive waste in the body or even excessive fluids in the body that is brought by unburned fat. Some of the signs to know that you are suffering from kidney failure are like of appetite, itchy skin, or the urge of wanting to urinate more often.

- Cancer

Nobody likes the mention of cancer not now, not ever. Cancer is the leading source of death among most disease as most of the time, people get to know that they are suffering from it when it is too late and the doctors may not help much. Obesity is gear motivation of cancer in so many ways as it comes with various type of cancer. Some of these cancer brought around by obesity include the likes of pan creative cancer, breast cancer, or esophagus cancer.

Every problem is treated differently and the solution is never the same, the same applies to health. Apart from knowing the disadvantages that overweight may bring to the table, you ought to know all there is to discover the necessary solutions to be implemented. The 28 months loss program will help you lose weight and maintain a fitness program.

What is the proper meal plan for overweight?

In this section, you will be learning some of the tips to use and watch out for in order to reduce weight and in addition, examples of foods to eat to maintain your body and shape. Below are tips for weight loss known to have worked in all scenarios.

- ✓ Keep away from sugary foods like ice cream, yogurt, and chocolate milk among others.

- ✓ Ensure that you drink water before eating and probably an hour or so, which will help you not eat a lot.

- ✓ Make sure that in your meal plan, protein is the one dominating and carbohydrates are low.

- ✓ Lift weight to burn fat on your body.

✓ Keep in check the weight loss by measuring the body weight regularly for a positive attitude.

✓ Make sure that you have at least 8 hours sleep every day

✓ Be strict on your meal plan

Losing weight faster is determined by what is in your menu when it comes to the table. You might do exercise or follow the tips above, but the kind of foods you highlight on your table at the end of the day is meant to increase your body weight than actually reducing it.

The Proper Choice for Food and Meal Plan

The dash diet program mainly focuses on fruits and vegetables for the weight loss. A lot of people often question and ask if the diet program is meant to help everyone. Well, the answer to that is very simple, diet program helps everyone. The program aims to help those with obesity to lose weight and those with healthy bodies to maintain theirs.

Options for breakfast

Breakfast is defined differently by people depending on the beliefs and cultures of people. To some, it is advisable to eat heavy in the morning and lightly during lunchtime, while to others it is reverse light breakfast and heavy lunch.

For those suffering from overweight, the dash diet program advises them to go for the grains in the morning which are cereal foods too.

- ❖ Two slices of grain bread, mostly the one with wheat in it.
- ❖ Cereals
- ❖ White rice with tea

Selection for lunch

Lunchtime is something that should be considered strictly and watched out for as it determines your stomach for the rest of the day. Some people wake up late do breakfast and skip lunch, others do the opposite. The question is not the channel you choose for this approach, but proper routine to be considered for the program to be effective, therefore lunch is very important in this scenario.

The best selection is the simple organic option that entails vegetables and fruits.

- ❖ Green foods like spinach and cabbage or broccoli
- ❖ Fruit juice, at best pineapple and orange juice
- ❖ Fruit salad, try mixing fruits and eating them all together like avocados, orange, and watermelon.
- ❖ Grilled chicken
- ❖ Roasted vegetables

Appetizers

Appetizers can be used between lunchtime and supper. This can be boiled potatoes, small salad, or even tuna. Appetizers help the body prepare for the main course.

What to have for supper

Supper is often supposed to be a light meal to take in order to have a nice sleep. When the meal is taken in excessively, the night appears to be very long because the body won't allow you to have a nice sleep as digestion will still be taken place even in late night.

For the dash diet, the following are some of the best options to consider for your supper.

- ❖ Lean meat, chicken breast
- ❖ Smashed potatoes
- ❖ Brown rice
- ❖ Green peas
- ❖ Pork Fillet

Dash diet is very effective to the body and the result is ever awesome, the feeling will make you want to take pictures of yourself more often and even share the idea of the program to your fellow friends and family.

Dash diet is more effective when it is prompted by exercise after a meal than just focusing on the meal plan. There are some few regular yet simple and comfortable forms of exercises you can indulge for effective weight loss.

Running

Running is one of the best ways for health care as it helps to improve the physical and mental health of a person. Running is very important for all ages and health fitness regardless of suffering from something or not. Did you know that running reduces knee pain? Well, it does great, most of the overweight people suffer from knee pain caused by swollen knees. Therefore, this activity will bring the great impact of improving the knee pain. Running reduces weight loss fast whether it is outdoor running or treadmill running as it helps to burn calories and reduce fat in the body. Those suffering from depression will be helped in this area as running helps to set people in moods even after being stressed, as well as helps to improve aerobics activities on someone.

Hikes

Hiking was started out as recreation activity and was done for hobbies during free time. Today, hiking is not only used for a hobby, but also for a medical purpose. According to various researches, hiking has a great impact on weight loss and health maintenance. It helps in reducing problems associated with heart diseases. Improves the blood pressure level, hiking is also known to improve body balance and boost the body muscles.

Swimming

Swimming is a great sport for health care as it requires people to use all their body parts for effectiveness. This ensures that muscles are built stronger and the heart makes sure that oxygen is generated well in all parts of the body. Is swimming a good way of reducing weight? Yes, it does contribute a lot in this section and the body gets to relax at the end of the day.

Most of those suffering from overweight often seem not to do anything in the house but to just eat and watch or engage in online games. Housework activities are a very important exercise for weight loss and the body. Housework not only burns calories through the efforts needed but also help someone to reduce stress by engaging in these activities as the mind gets to be distracted from the bother it had encountered.

Those are the outdoor activities that are important and enact a great change in people, probably the best for beginners. Obesity to beginners is very hectic as they find very hard to cope with situations as they are enclosed in a completely different world, thus change is impeccable. For beginners, I would recommend to be strict with these tips and solutions and observe every change that happens to them. Some are advised to reduce the amount of salt intake in the body which is good, though excessive reduction of salt intake by itself is a danger as it leads to blood pressure.

Apart from the outdoor activities of exercise, there are also indoor activities which are also very effective to weight loss, is monitored well, and they should undergo a certain regular routine, basically at least 2 times a day. When it comes to exercise, strict rules are followed and there are channels to be used first before beginning this exercise; they are like deserts. Before using the weights, you should do basic exercises first for your body in order for the muscles to be prepared for the heavy lifting.

Basics before Lifting Weights

Squats

Squats are very important to the body especially when it comes to muscles on the hips. Squats are simply done through frequent leaning and getting up. According to the exercise, the leaner you do, the more muscle mass you will have. Squats prepare the legs for heavy lifts like the dead pull which requires a lot of energy from the legs.

Pull ups and push ups

This is another basic necessity before using the weights. When you do the pushups and pull-ups, the body increases the stamina or the muscles, generally the biceps and triceps, making using weight not tire the body fast, but keep up with the strength.

Treadmill

This is an indoor activity that involves running or jogging on a moving metal. Its aim is burning calories fat within a short time. The best advantage of the treadmill is the fact that you can set the speed you want to run. For beginners, it is well advised to start with low speeds then move up slowly until the body is able to balance and keep up with the speed. Other than that, treadmill is most prepared because even in a hurry to go somewhere else, that short time is enough to trigger a change in your body.

How to Start Weightlifting for Beginners

It is believed that weights were started to increase mass and were aimed for the men only according to statics on most people. Weights are not just for increasing the mass in muscles but to keep fit and reduce weight loss for both men and women.

Most beginners suffering from overweight find it challenging when they enter the gym for the first time on where to start and how to start in order to reduce weight. Don't worry about any of them anymore, this section will help you through all that.

There are some few tips to consider first before enrolling in the weights:

✓ Know what each weight is meant for

✓ Don't go for the heavyweights first

✓ Ask on anything you are not sure before acting

✓ Ask for help during lifting weights

✓ Always carry water to the gym

With that, you are good to go, you can now start lifting your weights.

Why is there no change after going to the gym?

This question is frequently asked a lot, especially by the beginners, as they try out everything to see into it that their weight loss is effective. Well, everything requires time and commitment, and most importantly, they require patience. As a beginner, don't ever expect to go to the gym for one month and expect that there will be a massive change in your body. At times, you might not see any change yourself but those around you can monitor a great change in that one month in you.

Below is a list of reasons why there is no change in your weight after hitting the gym for a month.

a) Lifting the very lightweight

b) The wrong plan meal

c) Wasting a lot of time in the gym doing other things rather than workout

d) Doing the lifts the wrong way

e) Being lazy and going to the gym twice a week instead of twice a day

f) Not changing your workout routine and doing it every day
g) Mixing all the work out at the same time indulges very little change in the body
h) Holding the weights the wrong way
i) Eating a lot of calories before the gym

For effective weight loss on the dash diet program, there are don'ts when it comes to choice of food or the body will continue being fatter. Some of the examples of don'ts when it comes to choice of food while on the diet is cheese, red meat, and fried foods. They contain a lot of calories and they need to be watched out. It is with this sort of foods that there is an increase in diseases during overweight and they are at times hectic to cure. At times, the doctor may find the patients having more diseases at a go and treating them all together is never easy.

Chapter 4: Your General Health with the DASH Diet Approach

What do you understand by dieting and who should diet? What do you think dieting entails? Well, if you are like most people, you must associate dieting with losing weight or a meal plan followed by the sick. Dieting, and more so the Dash diet approach, is for every person aspiring to have a healthier lifestyle regardless of their body size or shape, gender, or age. Everyone desires to live a healthier life free from lifestyle diseases hence the holistic approach to healthier living through the Dash Diet.

Importance of Healthy Eating Habits

Life is about bargains, isn't that so? Indeed, in the event that you want to disregard your terrible dietary patterns that you practice routinely, reconsider. A mistake that numerous individuals make is imagining that on the off chance that you burn off a huge amount of calories at the gym, you can eat anything you desire. Or on the other hand, in case you are naturally thin, you don't need to watch what you eat. Shockingly, exchanging an hour in the gym for an oily twofold cheeseburger or depending on a decent metabolism to replace smart dieting propensities totally overlooks the main issue of carrying on with a sound way of life.

Healthy eating is not an easy affair. This is because human beings base their food choices on their taste rather than their nutritional value. A lot of times, we overeat on the unhealthy foods because they taste good and end up feeling bad because we are aware of the damage we have caused our bodies. The unhealthy food choices are also readily available and affordable, making it an easier alternative for many.

To understand the importance of healthy eating, we must begin by understanding why we eat as human beings. Human beings need to eat in order to supply their bodies with nutrients found in carbohydrates, Vitamins, Proteins, Minerals, and fats. The basic need for food is to fuel the body for its daily functions. Just like a car needs the right kind of fuel to function properly, the human body also needs the right kind of food to fuel it; wrong food will cause damage to the body.

Healthy eating is not easy. It requires sacrifice and a lot of discipline. But if it is so hard, why bother? Well, at one point in your life, you will realize that your health determines the kind of lifestyle you will lead. As a person picks up smoking habit, they are faced with the realization that they may get lung cancer or any respiratory diseases owing to their lifestyle. This is the same thinking that a person that does not choose healthier eating habits should have. If one wants to live a long and healthy life, they must therefore make decisions to healthy eating habits.

It is unfortunate that majority of the people do not have time or the will power to invest in healthier lifestyles. Unhealthy eating and lifestyles have become the norm due to the busy schedules of our daily lives.

Common Unhealthy Eating habits

Almost everyone in one way or another has practiced unhealthy eating and lifestyle habits. Some of the common ones are as listed below:

1) Skipping breakfast - Generally, it is known as the most essential meal of the day and skipping it can prompt metabolic slump.
2) Drinking excessive liquor – A lot of alcohol can trigger weariness and hypertension
3) Smoking – Smoking is likely to bring with it heart problems, breathing complications, and even lung cancer as well as mouth cancer
4) Lack of a balanced diet meal - Excessively low-quality diet can cause weight gain and the taking of sugary beverages can raise the danger of diabetes.
5) Overeating – Excessive eating can cause undesirable weight gain and hypertension

6) Sedentary Lifestyle – Lack of any physical activity can lead to excessive weight and a weak heart.

7) Not drinking enough water – Lack of drinking enough water will lead to dehydration and poor digestion.

Effects of Unhealthy Eating – Fast Foods

With the fast-paced lifestyles many people are faced with, healthy eating has become non-existent with many turning to fast foods that are known to cause many problems in the human body. Some of the effects of this unhealthy lifestyle include;

- Headaches – High sodium foods like fast foods increase the risk of headaches
- Depression – studies show that increased consumption of processed and fast foods can lead to depression.
- Dental distress – Carbs and sugar produce acids that can destroy the teeth enamel
- Acne – Carb heavy foods like French fries trigger acne breakouts
- Shortness of breath – Extra calories turn to extra pounds hence obesity causing shortness of breath and wheezing
- Heart Disease – Elevated cholesterol levels increase blood pressure leading to heart disease.
- High Cholesterol – Fried foods are high in trans fats that raise bad cholesterol.

- Blood pressure – Fast foods are high in sodium which is likely to elevate blood pressure
- Weight gain – The number of calories found in fast foods is too high leading to obesity
- Blood sugar spike – Fast foods are filled with empty carbohydrates causing frequent insulin spikes
- Bloating and puffiness – The body is likely to retain water due to the high levels of sodium in fast foods leaving one feeling puffy and swollen.
- Insulin resistance – Fast foods can lead to insulin fluctuations and resistance resulting in type 2 diabetes.

Effects of Unhealthy Eating to the Cardiovascular System

Most drive-thru foods which include sides and beverages are extremely high in sugars with next to zero fiber. When your stomach related framework breaks up these substances, the carbs are converted as glucose (sugar) into your circulation system. Thus, the increase in glucose. The pancreas will react to the flood in glucose by releasing insulin. Insulin moves the sugar on the entire body to cells which require it for vitality. Your glucose comes back to typical, as your body uses or stores the sugar.

This procedure in glucose is managed by your body, and insofar as you're sound, your organs can appropriately deal with these spikes in sugar. Be that as it may, often eating foods that are rich in carbs can trigger rehashed spikes in your glucose. After some time, these spikes in insulin can cause your body's ordinary insulin reaction to flounder. This builds your hazard for insulin opposition, type 2 diabetes, and weight gain.

Effects of Excessive Sodium to the Body

To a few people, the mix of sugar, fat, and loads of salt can make drive-thru foods more delectable. That being said, consuming fewer calories high in sodium can prompt water maintenance, the very reason you may feel swollen, enlarged, or puffy after eating drive-thru food. For individuals with circulatory strain conditions, an eating regimen high in sodium is additionally unsafe. Sodium can hoist circulatory strain and add weight on the cardiovascular framework and the heart.

Around 90% of grown-ups disparage the amount of sodium that is in their drive-thru food dinners as indicated by one investigation. The examination overviewed 993 grown-ups and found that their speculations were multiple times lower than the genuine number (1,292 milligrams). This, in essence, implies sodium levels were higher 1,000 mg.

Unhealthy Eating and the Nervous System

For the time being, cheap foods may fulfill hunger, however, long haul results are more negative. People that consume junk foods and prepared baked goods are 51% bound to suffer from depression than people who don't consume those nourishments or eat only a few of them.

Unhealthy Eating and the Respiratory System

Excess calories found in fast-food meals are associated with increased weight gain. This may lead to obesity. The extra weight can put pressure on your vital organs and symptoms may show up even with little trigger. You may notice difficulty in breathing when you're walking, climbing stairs, or exercising. In children, the risk of respiratory diseases is extremely evident. One study found that those that ate fast food at least thrice a week were more likely to develop asthma.

Effects of Unhealthy Eating to the Skeletal System

Carbs and sugar in junk food and prepared sustenance can expand acids in your mouth. These acids can separate tooth enamel. As tooth enamel vanishes, microbes can grab hold and holes may create. Heftiness can likewise prompt inconveniences with bone thickness and bulk. Individuals who are stout have a more serious hazard for falling and breaking bones. It's essential to continue practicing to fabricate muscles, which bolster your bones and keep up a solid eating regimen to limit bone misfortune.

Effects of Unhealthy Eating to the Society

Today, more than 2 of every 3 grown-ups in the United States are viewed as overweight. More than 33% of youngsters ages 6 to 19 are likewise viewed as overweight.

The development of junk food in America appears to match with the development of weight in the United States. The Obesity Action Coalition (OAC) reports that the quantity of drive-thru food eateries in America has multiplied since 1970. The quantity of hefty Americans has likewise dramatically increased. In spite of endeavors to bring issues to light and make Americans more brilliant customers, one examination found that the measure of calories, fat, and sodium in cheap food suppers remains to a great extent unaltered.

As people get busier and eat out more often as possible, it could have unfavorable impacts for the individual and the social insurance framework.

What is then the alternative to unhealthy eating habits?

Unhealthy lifestyles or eating habits have become such a worrying phenomenon with government and health practitioners leading to the development of guidelines to healthier eating like the Dash Diet Approach. If people took the discipline to change their lives and adopt healthier ways of

49

eating, the above discussed negative effects of unhealthy eating on people will not be faced.

There are many benefits to healthy eating as highlighted below

- More productive – When you eat right, the brain and body get the right amount of fuel, hence increased productivity. Some foods are also very good at preventing some diseases. If one eats fatty fish and a lot of vegetables, they prevent diseases like Alzheimer or dementia.
- A happier self – Some foods affect ones' mood. A lot of fatty foods are likely to make one sluggish and put you in a bad mood. Bananas and small amounts of dark chocolate are known to be great mood boosters.
- Stress Reduction – Studies have shown that eating foods rich in proteins reduce the body levels of cortisol, a stress hormone.
- Saving money – Healthy eating eventually saves money. This is because you will not spend on medical bills caused by lifestyle diseases.
- Weight Control – There are many lifestyle diseases associated with obesity. When one chooses a healthy eating lifestyle, body weight is controlled hence diseases are kept at bay.
- Developing a healthy food plate – The healthier the food you eat, the more you will appreciate the taste and crave it more as opposed to unhealthy food choices.

- Staying Younger – Vegetables and fruits are high in antioxidants helping protect and improve your skin. One looks younger for longer.
- Live longer – With the threat of lifestyle diseases dealt with, one is more likely to live longer and die a natural death not one out of diseases.
- Controlled portion – Healthy food options do not give one the craving to eat more food than the body requires. This ensures a calorie controlled diet.
- A healthier heart – There are many factors that increase the risk of heart diseases. Diet is one of the major factors. Healthy and balanced diet plan greatly reduces the risk of heart diseases.
- Better cholesterol levels – Cholesterol is the fat that clogs a person's arteries. A controlled healthy diet with lots of vegetables ensures controlled cholesterol in the blood.
- Strong Immune System – Foods rich in vitamins are known to improve the immune system. A healthy diet includes a lot of vegetables and fruits that are rich in vitamins that help fight diseases.
- Better Sexual function – Studies have linked unhealthy eating to lower libido in both men and women. Too much fat in the body causes some of these bodily functions to slug.
- Improved sleep – Overeating leading to obesity causes unhealthy sleeping patterns and has been linked to causes of insomnia.

Why the Dash Diet Approach as Compared to Other Diets in the Market

According to Wikipedia, the Dietary Approach to Stop Hypertension or commonly known as DASH diet has consistently been ranked as a top diet for a healthy heart and weight loss. The Dash diet is not a fad diet. It has been supported by scientific evidence that backs its efficacy and involves controlled and manageable dietary changes that are flexible and based on proven nutritional advice. This has made it a preferred choice by doctors and other health practitioners to their patients.

The Dash diet plan was developed specifically to help people lower high blood pressure. There are many food options in this diet with a focus on whole foods such as fruits and vegetables, low-fat and fat-free dairy, lean meats like white meat, and whole grains. This plan also focuses on eliminating or limiting consumption of processed foods, sugary drinks, packed snacks, as well as red meat that has been associated with high levels of saturated fats.

The Dash diet is also centered on low sodium (salt) requirements thus reducing water retention thus giving an advantage over hypertension. This diet is highly recommended for people that come from families with a history of heart disease or those at risk of type 2 diabetes and also helps these conditions on people with the diseases already.

Types of DASH Diet

There are 2 main types or forms of DASH diet namely The Standard Dash diet that controls the daily sodium intake to 2,300 milligrams and the Lower-Sodium Dash diet that limits daily consumption of sodium to 1,500 milligrams. Depending on one's health needs, one can choose from any of the two diet plans. On average, the daily Dash diet meal plan involves the following:

- Six to eight servings of whole grains
- 6 or fewer servings of meat preferably poultry and fish
- 4 to 5 servings of vegetables preferably green leafy ones
- 4 to 5 servings of fresh fruit not canned
- 2 to 3 servings low-fat dairy and if watching weight, then fat-free dairy
- 2 to 3 servings of healthy fats like avocado oils, coconut oils, or olive oils

The nutritional goals expected from the above plan are:

- Fat should be 27% of calories consumed
- Not more than 6% of calories in saturated fats
- Proteins constitute 18% of calories consumed
- Carbohydrates take the biggest percentage at 55% of the calories
- Cholesterol from the diet should not exceed 150mg
- 30 grams or more of fiber is expected

Depending on ones' weight or the need to weight loss, one can choose a diet plan that provides 1,200, 1.400, 1,600, 1,800, 2,000, 2,600 or more calories per day.

How the Dash Diet Works to Lower Blood Pressure

This diet is centered along controlling salt intake as well as limiting consumption of cholesterol and saturated fats, both of which are high contributors to heart diseases. It also focuses on increasing the taking of whole grains and fresh fruits resulting in effective results while following this diet plan. It is highly recommended that those using it must combine it with other healthy lifestyle approaches like exercising, losing weight, reducing alcohol consumption, and possibly stop smoking altogether.

Benefits of the DASH Diet Approach

Although this diet was originally developed for persons desiring to lower their blood pressure, over time, it has also been seen as a great option to those that seek to adopt a healthier lifestyle or diet. It emphasizes on consuming whole foods that have low percentage of unhealthy fats and added sugars, as well as controlled portions leading to weight loss. Some of the benefits of following this diet plan include the following:

- Long-Term Potential – what this simply means is that the diet has a lot of food options and one is not likely to run out of food options while on the program.
- Lower Blood Pressure and Cholesterol levels – It is a well-documented fact that heart diseases are among the top killers over the world. Lowering blood pressure and cholesterol levels minimize to a great deal the chances of heart diseases.
- Reduces risk of other diseases – Following a Dash diet is likely to reduce the risk of a stroke. A strong heart also results in improvements of other bodily functions like kidney functions, blood sugar management, and eye health.
- Better Management of type 2 Diabetes – When paired with an exercise plan and a weight loss plan, the Dash diet has been found to reduce insulin resistance which is the cause of type 2 diabetes.
- Better Nutrition – The Dash diet emphasizes on eating of whole and fresh foods as opposed to processed and pre-packed foods that are full of added salt and sugar.

How to Start the Dash Diet

This diet calls for several small servings of food daily from various food groups. These servings, however, do vary depending on the number of calories needed by the individual per day. The Dash diet is a combination of all food categories. It is rich in low-fat dairy foods, vegetables, fruits, and low saturated fats as well as cholesterol. It is high in dietary fiber, magnesium, calcium, potassium, and moderate proteins.

This diet plan calls for gradual changes to ones' eating habits as drastic changes have overtime proved to be detrimental to ones' health instead. For instance, start by limiting your daily intake of sodium to about one teaspoon. Once your body adjusts, cut back to three-quarters of a teaspoon until you get to desired levels.

Customize Your Diet to more Dash-Like

The Dash diet has no set foods, just guidelines. By doing the following, one can therefore adapt their current diet to the Dash guidelines.

- Consume more fresh fruits and vegetables
- Substitute refined grains for whole grains
- Opt for fat-free, low-fat or skimmed dairy products
- Opt for lean proteins like fish, chicken, or plant protein like beans
- Only use healthy vegetable oils while cooking
- Reduce intake of sugar-filled foods like candy or processed drinks
- Reduce consumption of foods that are saturated in fats such as oils, full-fat dairy, and meat.

- Opt more on low-calorie drinks like water, herbal teas, and coffee

The Dash Diet Approach for Vegetarians and Vegans

The Dash diet is also suitable for Vegetarians and Vegans alike. With some tweaking of the plan by using substitutes of meats, dairy, and eggs, the Dash diet can be beneficial to both vegans and vegetarians. One needs to substitute these products with soy-based products and plant-based proteins while following the set guidelines of the Dash diet approach.

Frequently Asked Questions

Just like any other type of diet out there, a person wishing to adopt the Dash diet plan approach is likely to have many questions. It is important to ask questions as it reduces the ambiguity surrounding the plan and enables one to follow it accurately. Some of the most asked questions include:

1) **Can I take coffee or other caffeinated drinks?**
   With this diet, there are no specified guidelines for drinking coffee or other caffeinated drinks. However, it is a well-documented fact that caffeinated drinks such as coffee may lead to a short-term spike in blood pressure. A recent study however claims that coffee doesn't

increase long-term risks of hypertension or heart disease. For people with normal blood pressure however are said that they can safely take 3 to 4 regular cups of coffee a day. Those with high blood pressure are however advised to minimize the intake of caffeine.

2) Must I exercise while on the Dash diet?
Studies have shown that physical exercise paired with a healthy diet lowers blood pressure more than diet alone. It is recommended to do 30 minutes of moderate exercise like brisk walking, jogging, swimming, cycling, and even housework to see great results.

3) Can I take alcohol on the Dash diet?
Excessive drinking has been linked with increased blood pressure. Regular drinking of more than 3 drinks a day has been associated with various heart diseases. While on the Dash diet, one should take alcohol sparingly and must not exceed official guidelines of 2 drinks a day for men and 1 drink for women.

The only answer to a healthier lifestyle devoid of diseases is to adopt a healthier way of eating. The Dash Diet Approach provides an easier guide to alternative eating that is affordable to all and will lead to greater health for the majority. The world is plagued by lifestyle diseases that have brought down life expectancy as many people die prematurely due to poor health.

If many people adopt the Dash Diet Approach, lifestyle diseases will be a thing of the past and hence creating healthier nations.

Chapter 5: Steps towards Transitioning to the DASH Diet

You've decided to transition to a DASH diet (Dietary Approaches to Stop Hypertension). You already know its benefits but where do you begin? Worry no more. I am about to give you steps in which you can transition to a DASH diet correctly. The true test and the biggest question I'll have for you is this, "Will you stick to the diet"? You certainly can and this shouldn't hinder you from going forward with it. As they say, the hardest part of a journey is taking the first step. From then on, you look back and you'll be amazed at just how much you've achieved. This is because the DASH diet is not rocket science, and getting the ingredients and preparing meals is something that can easily be done. The best part about it is that you are not completely throwing away your daily menu but you are incorporating the DASH diet into your menu. Some days you'll feel like eating more and other days less for a particular food category. That's totally okay, as long as you don't steer so much from the recommendations. The only thing that doctors give as an exception is sodium. It is highly advisable not to exceed the limit for sodium.

As you get started on the DASH diet, kindly unlearn the following misconceptions and also teach the people around you about it. This would even go a long way by having people to support you and hold you accountable along the way.

- **The DASH diet is only for individuals with high blood pressure** - while the diet helps individuals that have high blood pressure, they are not the only ones who need to be concerned with what they are taking. Something like exceeding the limits of sodium intake can take a toll on anyone's body.

- **The sole focus of a DASH diet is low sodium or no salt** - Sodium reduction is a recommendation, but not the only one. Other nutrients which play a role in good health are recommended.

- **The DASH diet is an "all or nothing diet"**- this is a common misconception that holds people from transitioning to a DASH diet. Many people are scared of starting the plan for fear of failing and having side effects after returning to old eating habits. The diet is all about incorporating better food choices to your meal plans which are realistic and achievable.

Let's begin with what is your aim in the whole transitioning to the DASH diet.

These are the things you want to eat more:

- Nuts
- Fruits
- Low-fat or Fat-Free Dairy
- Whole grains
- Vegetables
- Lean Meat, Fish, and Poultry.

Foods that you will eat less or totally eliminate

- Sodium
- Fatty meats
- Saturated and Trans Fats
- Sugar and Sweets

Keep in mind that you don't want to transition to the diet all at once. As you introduce new foods, especially those rich in fiber, your digestion may change. You'll want to slowly and gradually incorporate them into your meal plans until it now becomes a routine. The changes could be over a couple of days or even weeks. Because a DASH diet has high fiber, fluid intake should be increased at the same time. Fiber tends to draw water into the bowel which could lead to hard stool and constipation. Also, as you begin on the DASH diet, clean out your cabinet. Those sugary, salts, and snacks that might tempt you in the future. Donate the food to a local food bank. Another key thing to note on the DASH diet is that you'll limit the number of times you eat out. The amount of sugar, fats, and oils in a restaurant is almost impossible to know.

Steps to note while transitioning to the DASH diet

1. Maintain a food diary

This could be an app or just a physical diary. In this diary is where you record the changes you see in addition to having goals that you set on a daily basis. This gives you a sense of accountability and can also be used if there is a need to see a doctor.

2. Do not skip meals

The DASH diet includes a minimum of three meals. Don't skip lunch and then say you'll make up for it in the evening.

3. Be cautious with the food labels

You are heavily fighting sodium in this diet. When shopping, read labels. Here's the secret. If a label says "reduced sodium", run for your dear life. Reduced sodium does not mean its low. Low sodium diet has 140mg of sodium per serving. The recommended daily sodium intake per day is less than 2,300 mg.

4. Taking note on daily servings

Here's the thing, a serving will be unique to you based on the following metric. The number of calories you should be healthily taking each day. How will you estimate the calorie intake? This will be based on your age, gender, and the kind of work you do. There are various apps you can use on the internet to guide you on the right amount of calories you should be consuming. Keep a record to monitor your success.

5. Compare DASH with your current meal menus

Depending on your eating patterns, choose to either increase or decrease your food portions.

6. Begin on the DASH diet

Being equipped with information about a DASH diet is not enough. Start working on it. The key is to plan ahead and stock your kitchen with the DASH foods. Based on your meal plan, create a meal plan to make a better decision with your shopping list.

Creating a Meal Plan

The meal plan should be made with the following eating times in mind at a minimum.

1. Breakfast

2. Lunch

3. Dinner.

Keep the following in mind while and before shopping.

1. **Don't shop when hungry** - You know those foods especially fast food and the sugary foods that you can't resist yourself from eating? Well, the desire to eat them is very high when hungry. So eat first before you go to a shop.

2. **Read the labels** - For packaged food, read their nutrition labels. Be extra keen on the fat and sodium as earlier stated.

3. **Less packaged and fresher food** - Instead of going for canned fruits, go for the fresh ones. The same case applies to vegetables. The fresh foods in most cases still have their original nutrients and therefore more health promoting.

Breakfast options

As earlier stated, the DASH diet doesn't have a specific list of food to eat. The key thing is per serving to serve different food groups. The following breakfast shopping list will enable you to try different DASH breakfast recipe meals found on the internet and cookbooks.

- Whole-wheat bread
- Eggs
- Bananas
- Low-fat milk
- Oatmeal

- Peanut butter
- Yogurt
- Cranberry juice
- Trans-free margarine
- Skim milk
- Strawberries or raspberries

Lunch list

- Green vegetables like Spinach, Kales, Broccoli
- Almonds
- Carrots
- Fruits such as melons, apricots, dates, grapes, mangoes, tangerines, and blueberries
- Turkey
- Whole-grain crackers

Dinner

- Olive oil
- Whole wheat spaghetti
- Beef
- Wild rice
- Chicken
- Tuna
- Broccoli
- Potatoes

- Green peas

Narrowing down to the individual food groups

➢ **Whole grains** - sources of whole grains include whole-grain bread, whole-grain cereals, brown rice, oatmeal

➢ **Vegetables** - vegetables can go up to 4 servings per day. It includes leafy green vegetables like kales and spinach. Other good sources include broccoli, carrot and tomatoes, Brussels sprouts, and sweet potatoes. They are packed with high fiber, potassium, magnesium, and healthy vitamins. Both raw and cooked vegetables work well. Avoid frozen vegetables.

➢ **Fruits** - also up to 4 serving per day. The DASH diet includes eating a lot of fruits. This could be from apples, pineapples, grapes and berries, peaches, and mangoes. It is highly recommended that you eat edible peels of fruits such as apples and pears. The peels contain healthy nutrients and fiber. Fruits can be enjoyed as a side dish with other meals or as a snack. If you have to buy canned fruit, check the label for added sugar which should be avoided. Fruits such as grapefruit can clash with certain medications so it is advisable to consult your doctor or a pharmacist before then

➢ **Dairy Products** - could go up to 3 servings per day. Dairy products in the DASH diet should have low fat since dairy can be loaded with fat. Low-fat cheese, low-fat yogurt, and skim milk. Consult the doctor if you are lactose intolerant or have a hard time digesting dairy. They will most probably describe pills that can aid in digestion and reduce the effects of dairy intolerance.

➢ **Fish, Meat, and Lean Chicken** - 5 or fewer helpings a day. Be keen to reduce on red meat and increase more white meat. Tuna and salmon have omega-3 fatty acids which lower cholesterol. What does one serving of meat look like? Well, the area of your palm could well guide you on this. An average palms estimate is 3 ounces. Avoid fatty meat such as bacon. Also, take away the fat and skin from poultry and meat. If possible bake, grill, or broil meat instead of frying.

➢ **Legumes, seeds, grains, and nuts** - these include walnuts, peanuts, peas, lentils, rice, pasta, sunflower seeds, and kidney beans. These could go up to 4 or 5 servings per week. The serving size for these foods is rather small because they contain high-fat content and a lot of calories.

Look for whole-grain bread which has more nutrients compared to refined grains. Be on the lookout for products labeled "100 percent whole wheat'. Also, learn to enjoy grains without adding things such as butter or cheese which have fat. For a nice crunch, you can try sprinkling them on salads. Soybean-based products are good alternatives to meat because just like meat, they contain all amino acids required by the body to make a complete protein.

- ➢ **Oils and fats** - the choice oils matter a lot. Too much fat increases one's chances of heart disease, diabetes, and obesity. Just to clarify, fat isn't necessarily a bad thing. It actually helps your immune system. The key thing is to avoid trans fats in fried and processed foods. Saturated fat is also a key culprit in increasing the risk of coronary artery disease. The DASH diet highly recommends vegetable oils. Corn oil, olive oil, and canola oil. Read labels on things such as margarine to select those that are trans-fat-free and low amounts of saturated fats.

- ➢ **Sugar** - cutting on sugar all at once might be a difficult task. The alternative thing is to use things like honey, agave syrup, and maple syrup in extremely limited quantities. You can sneak something like a diet cola in your meals, but it shouldn't be a substitute for plain water. Cut back on added sugar, which only adds calories and has no nutritional value.

> **Sweets** - these go up to 5 servings or fewer a week. DASH diet isn't harsh. It doesn't tell you to banish sweets all at once. It advises you to go easy on them by choosing those that are fat-free or low fat.

The above was just to get you started on the DASH diet. They are not the only foods but it's wise to use the following guidelines and tips.

- ✓ Reduce or limit the intake of sugary foods and beverages.
- ✓ Use vegetable oils to cook
- ✓ More white meat, less red meat
- ✓ Low-fat or fat-free dairy products
- ✓ Be careful and observant with sodium in food labels
- ✓ Measured fresh fruit juice portions
- ✓ Drinking alcohol sparingly and coffee in moderation. The recommended amount of alcohol in women is a maximum of 1 drink per day or less and men a maximum of 2 drinks per day or less
- ✓ Use herbs, spices, and things to enhance flavor instead of adding salt
- ✓ If you have to buy canned food, kindly rinse food such as beans to wash away excess salt
- ✓ You can substitute things like sugar with honey during baking or beverage drinks

- ✓ Serve fruits as snacks
- ✓ Reduce salad dressing

If you have other medical condition, it is wise to see a doctor who will help you in having a personalized DASH diet to meet your goals without medically harming yourself.

Incorporating Physical Exercise to the DASH Diet

Exercises with the DASH diet will to no surprise yield even more benefits. Exercising on its own has its benefits. Imagine now doing it together with the DASH diet. The DASH diet in all its moderation will not require you to go to do high intensive exercises. Do something you enjoy and moderate activity.

Some of the moderate activity you could do is cycling, walking, swimming, house chores, and light aerobics.

The recommended amount is at least 2hrs and 30 minutes per week of activities at moderate intensity. Gradually increase to 5 hours per week.

Utensils and Cookware

Equipping yourself with the right kitchen equipment helps in preparing and to follow through the DASH diet.

- ➢ Using non-stick cookware keeps the food from sticking and is easy to clean. Nonstick pans do not get affected with the browning that uncoated stainless pans get, hence you end up preparing a healthier meal.

> It has been proved through health-conscious cooks that they use less oil with nonstick cookware compared to uncoated cookware.

> Non-stick cookware also evenly distributes heat which is very important in cooking food faster.

> Moreover, non-stick cookware looks stylish and modern making it more appealing while cooking your DASH diet.

Overall, there is a misconception that a DASH diet leads to higher bills. The diet plan is easy to follow and plan. The DASH diet has actually been consistently ranked the best diet. This is because of its flexibility and how realistic it is. There are easy to find DASH diet recipes.

You could also try these money-saving tips.

1. If you have a backyard, grow your own food. It's not only fresh but also easily accessible, hence reduced excuses on a healthy meal.

2. Buy vegetables and fruits that are in season which most often have reduced prices compared to those not in season.

3. Choose generic brands.

To get the full benefits of the diet, don't look at it as a way to gain or lose weight. Keep it easy by just looking at it as a way in which you stay healthy. Otherwise, you might end up checking yourself in the mirror every now and then or measuring your weight every single time. The diet advises on about 2,000 calories a day. If your end goal is to lose weight, lower the number of calories while increasing the number of calories if the goal is to gain weight.

Most important thing is not to be so harsh on yourself. From time to time, reward yourself with a non-food treat for doing well with your accomplishment. Go for a movie, buy a book, or just do something for yourself. Celebrate small achievements which will lead to bigger achievements.

Chapter 6: What Should You Eat? What Shouldn't You Eat? The Do's and the Don'ts

Food this is one of the most loved topics. At the mention of food, most people smile because food is lovable - it causes excitement in the mind and to the body. Food is a basic necessity in life, something you can't leave without, something that should be done at least thrice in a day. That is a lot of topics to be discussed at the mention of food based on certain principles. Be it healthy, fitness, sweetness, or worst. This section will be focusing on the do's and don'ts of food, what to eat, and what not to eat.

What to Eat

Everyone loves food, like really a lot won't even complete a conversation with the mention of food. Especially those who love cooking, the food is everything. When it comes to what to eat, the topic is ambiguous, unless it is explained into small topics. The discussion is hard to break. The following are some of the major considerations that need to be observed considering what food to eat.

1. Health

74

2. Weight

3. Bodybuilding

4. Time

5. Disease Medication

6. Situation (pregnancy)

Every food has a purpose, people eat with different reasons and purpose objective.

Eating healthy

Eating healthy is very important, that is making sure that you are eating a balanced diet. That involves grains, vegetables, fruits, proteins, and foods rich in low fats. A person eating healthy is a person watching out for his/her body, someone who actually cares about how people view his/her body. This is a person who wants to look and feel good about the body. Healthy eating is eating food that is given prescription by the doctor. This is the foods that don't have excessive proteins or excessive calories but are all of the equal measures.

Healthy foods are categorized under different groups; the fats, proteins, carbohydrates, and fiber. Together in portions, they make a healthy result. Below is a list of some of the foods to be eaten in these categories and the portions to be taken in order to stay healthy.

Fats

This is foods that are rich in calories and should be definitely watched out for so as not to be eaten in excess. If the fats are eaten in excess, the result will be definitely obesity. Furthermore, obesity is not just bad but dangerous. It is a motivation of a lot of diseases.

Some examples of fats foods include:

❖ Yogurt cream
❖ Biscuits
❖ Cakes
❖ Fried foods
❖ Butter and margarine in bread

Fats in most cases are advised to be eaten in small portions for body safety.

Proteins

Proteins are the other food category that is highly valued in the body as they do most of the inner activities of the body like the regulation of both body and organ's tissue. Proteins are the source of food that should be dominating the most on the menu. They help in the development of bones and muscles in the body which are used in a lot of activities in everyday life. Most of the proteins are found in animal products.

Four reasons why you should put protein in your menu:

a) They are involved in repairing body tissues.

b) They help in fighting the body through diseases by the white blood cell.

c) They are involved in most transportation that takes place in the body.

d) The right amount of protein in the body is an assurance of the right growth and development of the baby or child and even for pregnant women.

Proteins are generally classified under four categories of structures.

- Primary structure
- Secondary structure
- Tertiary structure
- Quaternary structure

The four structures are determined by the DNA and RNA that are found in the body.

Examples of protein foods include the following:

❖ Baked beans
❖ Chapatti
❖ Meat
❖ Fish
❖ Eggs
❖ Cereal milk
❖ Legumes
❖ Red meat

Carbohydrates

This is food rich in molecules that are made up of three major sources: carbon, hydrogen, and oxygen. In some cases, they are also referred to as starchy foods.

Examples of carbohydrates include the following:

- ❖ Bread
- ❖ Rice both white and brown
- ❖ Potatoes
- ❖ Lean chicken pieces

Fiber

Fiber foods are also very important in this category and are eaten in great portions. This is a category of food that is prescribed by the doctor in great portion to be eaten in plenty. According to the current research that is observed in many situations, fiber comes with a lot of benefits. Like for instance, it prevents the body from filling empty and keeps it fuller most of the times. Apart from that, fiber is well known to reduce the chances of diabetes in the body as well as lowers the amount of cholesterol found in the body.

Examples of fiber include the following:

- ❖ Fruits
- ❖ Vegetables

- ❖ Whole grain breakfast
- ❖ Nuts
- ❖ Brown rice

The best tip of increasing fiber in fruits is by not peeling the skin off but instead wash it well and eat it as a whole.

Why eat healthily

Some people just eat healthy because it is recommended by the doctor but not because they know the importance of sticking to healthy foods.

Below are some of the reasons why you should eat healthily.

- ✓ Keeps you in good weight
- ✓ Makes you feel good about yourself
- ✓ Reduce diseases

Weight

Your body size determines a lot what you should or should not eat at all. A person trying to gain weight and a person trying to lose weight will definitely eat something very different at the end of the day. The one trying to increase weight will eat a lot of foods rich in calories, while the one trying to lose weight will make sure to reduce foods rich in calories in the menu and rather go for the vegetables.

What not to eat when trying to lose weight

- Sugary drinks
- Candy bars
- Ice cream
- Fried foods
- Cream in milk

Those are some of the foods that you should definitely watch out for and be very serious when it comes to them. If you dare try them out, you will be gaining more fat than losing weight. They may seem less harmful when you see them because they are very sweet but in reality, they motivate a lot in gearing up the calories in the body. Instead of them, I would recommend you go for less harmful types with less or zero calories in them. Try out the following list to your menu and within a month, there will be an impeccable change in your body.

- Lean meat, chicken breast
- Smashed potatoes
- Brown rice
- Green peas
- Pork Fillet

The above will not only help you reduce weight but keep you in very good shape.

According to the health station, for any change to be observed effective when it comes to losing weight, exercise is needed to boost up the changes and speed the process. For beginners, it is important not to just look for a proper diet as a method of losing weight, but also exercise as a method of speeding up the process.

These exercises can be indoors or outdoors. Some of the outdoors activities include running, swimming, hiking, and housework activities at the compound of the house. The indoors activates include squats, push-ups, press ups, weightlifting, and treadmill.

Importance of exercise for weight loss

a) Prevent diseases

There are so many diseases that come with obesity and some of them can be prevented by proper and regular exercises if done in the right way. Exercise helps to prevent heart diseases with activities like swimming. The exercises are important in burning up calories in the body, it helps to keep the body in balance especially with activities like hiking, and exercise sets the mood of a person and therefore ending up in reducing stress and depressions that may have occurred. Most of the overweight people suffer from swollen knees, therefore with the help of running exercise, improvement on the knees will definitely be seen.

b) Keeps the body fit

It is through these activities that the body is able to achieve balance by its own. Exercise makes people regain proper weight that is prescribed by the doctor and keeps them in the right shape. House chores are very important in initiating changes in the overweight as it requires efforts to move and pull things from one place to another. Exercises most of the time end up giving this person more muscles and fewer fats at the end of the day, if done well.

At times, people go to the gym and still not see any changes in their body because of not adhering to simple rules like:

a) Lifting the very lightweight
b) The wrong plan meal
c) Wasting a lot of time in the gym doing other things rather than workout
d) Doing the lifts the wrong way
e) Being lazy and going to the gym twice a week instead of twice a day
f) Not change your workout routine and doing it every day

As you can see, it is evident in this section that people at this level are not eating because they are hungry but instead they are eating because they want to reduce weight and keep in shape like other people. Overweight is one of the most dangerous encounters to ever have, it may even lead to death as it is well known to contribute to most of cancers diseases.

Bodybuilding

Foods that are rich in the development of bones and muscles, in most cases, they are proteins. This is the people who eat food because they want to increase mass in their body and become big. Proteins are therefore that kind of luxury, but again, be careful of the calories, you might overdo them and end up fat instead of fit. Some people might be tempted to try out calories and proteins because they speed up the process but they ought to know that it will always lead to being fat rather than fit because calories are known to dominate in most cases when misused.

Bodybuilding foods are mostly preferred by those doing jobs or work that require a lot of efforts like those that are working in constructions or queries. These people use a lot of efforts that drains their energy at the end of the day. Foods rich in proteins are more proper for them.

Time

Time is very essential when it comes to eating. Like the scriptures say, there is time for everything and everything should be done at the right time and not just randomly because it is supposed to be done.

What to eat is controlled by time under three distinctions: the breakfast, lunch, and supper. Every of this time has something that is recommended and according to the nutritionist, what you can eat at lunchtime is not what you should eat in the morning, everything with its own time. To some people, eating breakfast is not a must, they would prefer skipping it and eating heavy lunch instead. Well, there is no harm to that but the truth is all the three types of meals are very important and none should be skipped at all.

What to have for breakfast

This is one of the meals that have a history of being eaten in the wrong way. Most people don't know the proper meal plan for breakfast because they are not used to eat. Well, do not worry, I got your back on that. Below are some right choices preferred for breakfast in the morning.

- Eggs - according to most research, eggs is one of the most preferred meals in the morning and is used to help reduce blood sugar in the body especially the egg yolk.
- Greek yogurt - yogurt is rich in proteins and provides energy in the body. Yogurt is mostly preferred because they keep the stomach full for long before they feel empty again.
- Coffee - those who do or spent a lot of times in the office prefer coffee to tea mainly because coffee is well known to ensure that the body remains alert and the mood is often jovial.
- Nuts - nuts are not only sweet and tasty in nature, but they are also very important when it comes to

monitoring the body weight to ensure you don't get fat to obesity.

What to have for lunch

Some say breakfast is more important than lunch, some argue that the vice versa is true. Well, personally, don't let anyone fool you otherwise. Lunch is a very important part of the meal and is there mainly to help you get through the afternoon with a full stomach. Lunch is more effective especially when it is taken in the right way and in the right proportion. Below are some of the best options to consider for your lunchtime hour.

- Vegetables
- Sandwich
- Chicken salad
- Chips
- Black beans
- Potatoes

Lunch is important in various ways. For instance, lunch is important because it helps to increase the blood sugar during the day which results in concentration and alertness for the rest of the afternoon. Skipping lunch for those who take it likely should know that is very wrong and comes with severe consequences especially when you are working or a student. This is because when you skip lunch, chances of distractions and lots of attention in classes are very high which leads to poor performance at the end of the day.

What to have for supper

Supper is one of the hectic times in the meal plan and most people find it hard to stick to, especially the bachelors living alone. This is the people who leave for work early and return to the house late at night with tired bodies and mind. At this point, the mind is mostly tired and it just wants you to go to the shower, take a warm clean bath, and go to sleep till the next day. That occurs in a lot of times to most workers especially the low wage workers who are underpaid and work the most hours. Below are some simple foods you can prepare for your supper that get cooked and are ready within a short time.

- Spaghetti
- Beef stew
- Tuna and avocado
- Chicken bake
- scrambled eggs
- Broccoli

Those are some of the quickest foods to prepare for your supper within a short time before going to bed or if not in a hurry, you can try brown rice, fried meat, or fish.

Disease curing

Some people eat food for curing diseases as the main purpose at the end of the day. It is so true that these foods are not like the rest. I don't mean they taste different, but I mean they are situated in a very strict meal that ought to be followed under all situations in order to go well with the medicine provided by the doctor.

Fruits are mostly preferred in these situations especially the banana that helps in controlling the blood sugar level in the body. Yogurt is used to pushing medicine faster to the expected area, vegetable green foods like kales and spinach help to maintain the body and prevent weight gain at any time.

Situation

Some foods are taken based on certain situations and many of this time there is never otherwise of any alternative. It might be a prison form of situation, where you have to eat what other people are eating and there is no other option of selection, or it might be a pregnancy situation where a mother has to eat right in order to deliver a healthy baby when due.

Having known what to eat and when to eat and why to eat, we will then focus on the don'ts of what not to eat and the worst foods never to try in your menu as a concluding part.

What Not to Eat

✓ Microwave foods

The microwave is good for most people because they are fast to cook and save a lot of time to people especially those that prefer preparing quick foods. Well, that is good. It really helps a lot, but at the same time, the microwave is known to come with severe issues too. Like for instance, it may lead to diabetes or the fact that the food prepared is never evenly cooked.

✓ Hot dogs

It is true that they are very sweet and tasty and most people prefer buying them during sports activities or after running in the street. Hot dogs are junk foods and are rich in fats that lead to overweight if proper actions are not taken. The major danger that comes with it is the presence of sodium in them which is not needed in the body at all.

✓ Doughnuts

Doughnuts are the other sweet type of cakes that are loved by a lot of people because of their tasty allure. The sad truth is that these doughnuts are prepared by the GMO's which often leads to cancer when taken in excess and can even cause fast death from clogging the arteries.

- ✓ Pizza

  What is the first thing that comes to mind when you think of pizza? I don't know about you, but my first is that it is yummy. Pizza is the top in the list of the world eaten junk food with the most deliveries in a day. Most people love to order pizza during house parties or when left alone in the house by the parents or when there is no food in the house to eat and you are desperate for food in the stomach. Pizza is mixed with a lot of things that are rich in calories and that is the major reason why you should stop eating pizza from today.

- ✓ White bread

  Made from wheat white bread is a popular breakfast meal plan for a lot of people. I can't tell why people prefer white bread for breakfast but I can tell you why you should not eat white bread ever again. White bread is known to have low nutrients and is not good for the bodies, especially for the kids. A healthy kid must eat food rich in both nutrients and vitamins. The best alternative would be to go for the brown bread instead.

- ✓ Chips

  Many or almost everyone loves chips. They are very sweet and delicious, that smell by itself will increase your appetite from zero to hundred within seconds. Those who eat chips often will tell you how addictive chips are.

I wouldn't say chips are bad, but I wouldn't recommend them at the same time to anyone. Instead, I would recommend people to stop eating chips, this is because they have very high calories and the speed of increasing weight is very high and within three months of continuous eating, it may lead to overweight just like a joke.

✓ Ice cream

Talking of sweet things, ice cream is definitely on the list. It is an international thing that some people are very addicted that they would go a day with eating ice cream. I wouldn't say it is addictive, but I would say that taste will leave you craving for more when you are done. Ice cream is well-known to be rich in a lot of sugar which result in diseases like sugar level because the level of sugar that is put in the cream is in excess. Keep off ice cream for good and chances are that you wouldn't need to go to the doctor again to complain about your sugar level and waste a lot of money for regular checkups.

Some of these foods should only be good for the eyes and should not be there for the stomach. They are the kind of foods you should see in the restaurant and only ask for clean water, head home, cook, and eat healthily and also a balanced diet with no hurry. Foods are sweet, everybody knows that, but when the deal is too good, you must think twice. Not everything that glitters fits you, some should just be there for others and not you.

Chapter 7: Your Meal Plan for the Next 28 Days, Recipes You Can Use and What You Can Buy on Your Shopping List Each Week

Well, now that you have decided to take up the DASH diet, the next thing is to arm yourself with a meal plan. There are numerous books and recipes available to you online, hence getting a meal plan should not be a difficult thing for you.

This section features a simple meal plan you can follow for 28 days. It will guide you on what you should take every day for breakfast, lunch, and dinner. It will also feature the snacks you can take in between meals. You can rest assured that this meal plan will get you going with your DASH diet. So here we go.

Week 1

Day 1

Breakfast

Have hard-boiled eggs, a slice of bacon, and 6 ounces of low-sodium tomato juice. You can prepare several hard-boiled eggs and store them in the refrigerator for easy preparation.

Midmorning Snack

Baby carrots and a stick light cheese are an excellent choice for a midmorning snack.

Lunch

You can have quinoa meatless balls and cherry tomatoes. A side salad with vinegar dressing and a cup of Strawberry Jell-O will complete the meal perfectly.

Afternoon Snack

A handful of cashews and 4 ounces of lemon light yogurt

Dinner

Chicken Kabobs with salad and a cup of sugar-free raspberry Jell-O is good to complete the day.

Day 2

Breakfast

A fried omelet and 4-5 ounces of low-sodium tomato juice are good to start you off for the day.

Midmorning Snack

A cheese wedge slice and 6 grape tomatoes are enough for a light midmorning snack.

Lunch

Have 2 Turkey-Swiss roll-ups with cheese wrappings on the outside, a cup of coleslaw, and a cup of sugar-free Orange Jell-O for lunch.

Afternoon Snack

10 peanuts will be enough to keep you going until dinner time.

Dinner

For dinner, you can prepare roasted sliced turkey served with sautéed onions and carrot. Accompany the meal with a side salad and a cup of sugar-free Lime Jell-O.

Day 3

Breakfast

You can have scrambled eggs, a slice or two of Canadian bacon, and 4 ounces of cranberry juice.

Midmorning Snack

Your mid-morning snack could be made of 4 ounces of light low-fat yogurt and ¼ cup of almonds.

Lunch

Fried chicken breasts with no skin, coleslaw, and baby carrots will do for lunch. You can accompany the meal with a cup of lemon Jell-O.

Afternoon Snack

6 grape tomatoes and a slice cheese wedges.

Dinner

For dinner, go with a turkey burger, a cup of broccoli, and a side salad. Do not forget to finish with a cup or two of sugar-free strawberry Jell-O.

Day 4

Breakfast

Kick off your day with 8 ounces of skim milk, ¾ cup of Wheaties, and 4-6 ounces of raspberries or strawberries.

Midmorning Snack

The optional midmorning snack could be made of a light cheese wedge and grape tomatoes.

Lunch

For lunch, prepare 2-3 Swiss and turkey roll-ups accompanied by baby carrots and small plum.

Afternoon Snack

10 cashews and 6 ounces of blueberry yogurt should be more than enough for you.

Dinner

For dinner, you can have tilapia that has been pan-seared. In a skillet, heat a tablespoon of olive oil over medium-high heat and cook the tilapia, giving each side at least 4 minutes. The fish is ready when it flakes easily using a fork. You can coat the pieces with margarine or butter.

Accompany the fish with mango-melon salsa, fresh asparagus, and a cup of strawberry Jell-O.

Day 5

Breakfast

Hot chocolate, 2 hard-boiled eggs, and light cranberry juice will do for breakfast.

Midmorning Snack

10 ounces of almonds together with 6 ounces of lime yogurt will do just fine.

Lunch

Prepare a lunch made of Swiss and Turkey Sandwich. Put 3 ounces of turkey and a slice of Swiss cheese on two whole wheat bread slices then add tomato, lettuce, or any condiments of your choice. Pepper strips, Coleslaw, and Raspberry Jell-O cup complete the meal.

Afternoon Snack

Pepper strips and a half a cup of hummus.

Dinner

For dinner, you can prepare vegetable stir fry together with Quinoa. Add a fudge bar and a side salad with vinaigrette or Italian dressing.

Day 6

Breakfast

½ cup of cooked oatmeal, half a banana, 6 ounces of tomato juice and latte should get you going.

Midmorning Snack

Baby carrot and a stick light cheese are good for a midmorning snack.

Lunch

Three-Bean kale and brown rice served with sliced bell peppers are enough. Only add an Orange Jell-O cup.

Afternoon Snack

For snacks, you can have 10 cashews and 4-6 ounces of strawberries.

Dinner

For dinner, you can prepare white bean and some cabbage soup. Serve it with green beans, sliced tomatoes, and an Italian-dressed side salad. Complete the meal with a cup of nonfat, artificially sweetened, frozen yogurt topped with 4-6 ounces of raspberries.

Day 7

Breakfast

On the 7th day, you can have 1-3 scrambled eggs for breakfast accompanied by a slice of a light whole-wheat toast with a tablespoon of jam or jelly, 4 ounces of orange juice, and 8 ounces of skim milk or latte.

Midmorning Snack

4-6 ounces blueberries together with 10 almonds should be enough for a midmorning snack.

Lunch

Your lunch will be a bit heavier. 3 roast beef roll-ups and Muenster cheese together with Italian coleslaw and small peach make up the meal. Italian coleslaw is prepared just like the normal coleslaw, only that you add thin pepper strip, some grated carrots, and dressed with vinegar or oil.

Afternoon Snack

6 ounces of artificially sweetened strawberry light yogurt.

Dinner

For dinner, prepare salmon stuffed avocado, accompanied with a side salad and a low-fat bar of ice cream.

Week 2

Day 1

Breakfast

You can have egg toast with salsa. A toasted slice of whole-wheat bread, an egg, a pinch of pepper and salt and salsa are all you need to prepare this breakfast.

Midmorning Snack

Cinnamon pears will serve you well as a midmorning snack. Slice the pear and sprinkle cinnamon over the slices.

Lunch

Prepare a veggie-hummus sandwich for lunch. This simple snack carries 325 calories.

Afternoon Snack

For your afternoon snack, you can have ¾ cup of raspberries and any fruit juice.

Dinner

For dinner, you can prepare Lemmon-Herb salmon served with Caponata and Farro. A side salad and light, nonfat, yogurt completes the meal.

Day 2

Breakfast

For day two of the second week, you can prepare fig and honey yogurt for breakfast. You will need 2/3 cup nonfat, plain yogurt, 5 dried and chopped figs, 2 teaspoons of chia seeds, and 1 and ½ teaspoons of honey. The yogurt is prepared by simply topping the plain yogurt with the figs, honey, and chia seeds.

Midmorning Snack

Have yourself ½ a cup of grapes for a midmorning snack.

Lunch

For lunch, prepare white bean together with avocado salad. You will need two cups of mixed greens, ¾ cup of chopped vegetables, 1/3 cup of canned white beans, ½ avocado that has been diced, and 2 tablespoons of all-purpose vinaigrette. Top salad greens with the beans, avocado, veggies, and vinaigrette.

Afternoon Snack

Have yourself 1 clementine for the afternoon.

Dinner

You can prepare curried cauliflower steaks with Tzatziki and Red rice. Serve with nut and chocolate butter bites to make the meal tastier.

Day 3

Breakfast

A simple breakfast should do it for day 3 of week 2. Prepare a peanut butter cinnamon toast and latte to kick off your day.

Midmorning Snack

A cup of raspberries should complete your morning meal perfectly.

Lunch

Prepare a beef sandwich. Place a slice of well-fried beef, veggies, a slice of cheese, and any other sauce of your preference between two slices of whole-wheat bread. Add a cup of grapes to complete the meal.

Afternoon snack

Again, you can prepare cinnamon pears for your afternoon snack. Just as the previous time, slice the pear into pieces and sprinkle cinnamon on the pieces.

Dinner

For dinner, go for Mediterranean chicken served with Orzo salad. 1 clementine makes the meal even better. Preparing the chicken requires 2 chicken breasts, boneless, 3 tablespoons of olive oil, 1 teaspoon of lemon zest, ½ teaspoon of salt, ½ teaspoon of ground pepper, ¾ cup of whole-wheat orzo, 2 cups of sliced baby spinach, a cup of chopped cucumber, a cup of chopped tomato, ¼ cups of red onion, chopped, ¼ cup of crumbled feta cheese, 2 tablespoons of Kalamata olives, chopped, 2 tablespoons of lemon juice, and 1 clove of grated garlic.

To prepare, preheat the oven to 4250F. Brush the chicken with 1 tablespoon of oil. Sprinkle lemon zest, salt, and pepper. Bake for 30 minutes. Meanwhile, add a quart of water in a saucepan of medium size and boil over high heat. Add orzo and let it cook for 8 minutes before adding the spinach. Cook for a minute then drain. Use cold water to rinse before transferring the mix into a large bowl. Add the tomato, onion, feta, olives, and cucumber then stir to combine.

Day 4

Breakfast

A breakfast of yogurt and raspberries with nut will do it. You need a cup of plain yogurt, ½ a cup of raspberries, 5 chopped walnuts, and 1 tablespoon of honey. Simply top the yogurt with the other ingredients.

Midmorning Snack

Slices of a whole apple with cinnamon sprinkled on them is enough.

Lunch

For lunch, you can have a serving of white bean with avocado toast. A side salad of salad greens topped with carrots, cucumber, and vinaigrette complete the meal.

Afternoon Snack

1 medium plum

Dinner

You can have stuffed sweet potatoes dressed with a hummus dressing. You only need 1 large, scrubbed, sweet potato, ¾ cup of chopped kale, a cup of canned black beans, ½ cup of hummus, and 2 tablespoons of water.

Simply prick the sweet potato completely and microwave it for 10 minutes. In the meantime, place washed kales in a saucepan, cover and let it cook on medium-high heat. Once it has wilted, add bean, two tablespoons of water, and continue cooking for 2 minutes.

Split the sweet potato and top with the cooked mixture. Combine hummus in another dish with 2 tablespoons of water and drizzle the dressing over the sweet potato.

Day 5

Breakfast

For breakfast, prepare a peanut-butter cinnamon toast.

Midmorning Snack

2 clementines are enough to wrap up the morning meals.

Lunch

During lunchtime, you can prepare yourself a green salad with some pita bread and hummus. This meal requires you to top the greens with cucumber, carrot, and vinaigrette. This is then served with the pita bread and hummus. Complete the meal with a medium plum.

Afternoon Snack

A cup of grapes

Dinner

For dinner, you can prepare a main meal of chicken chili with sweet potatoes coupled with ¼ diced avocado and 1 tablespoon of nonfat plain yogurt. Top the chicken chili with the avocado and yogurt for a sweet meal.

Day 6

Breakfast

Start your day 6 with a fig and honey yogurt for breakfast. It is prepared by topping plain Greek yogurt with dried figs, 2 tablespoons of chia seed, and 1 ½ teaspoon of honey.

Midmorning Snack

A cup of raspberries will do just fine for your midmorning snack.

Lunch

For lunch, prepare Turkey with Pear Pita Melt. To prepare this, you will need ½ whole-wheat pita round, large, 3 ½ oz. deli turkey with low sodium levels, 1 sliced medium-sized pear, a tablespoon of shredded cheddar cheese, and a cup of mixed greens.

Use the turkey, cheese, and half the pear slices to stuff the pita pocket. Toast in an oven and add green onto the pita when serving. The remaining pear slices should be served on the side.

Afternoon Snack

1 medium plum

Dinner

A lemon-garlic shrimp served over orzo and zucchini is good for dinner. To make the dinner more enjoyable, add one clementine and a serving of nut and chocolate bites. This combination is enough to finish off your day without providing more sodium or calories than required.

Day 7

Breakfast

An egg toast with salsa is enough for breakfast. Simply top a slice of whole-wheat bread with egg, pepper, salt and salsa and your meal is ready.

Midmorning Snack

A banana

Lunch

Have chicken chili together with some sweet potatoes as prepared earlier this second week.

Afternoon Snack

½ cup of raspberries.

Dinner

For dinner, you can have chicken kabobs with salad and a cup of sugar-free raspberry Jell-O.

Week 3

Day 1

Breakfast

Your first breakfast of the week could be comprised of 1 bagel of whole wheat with 2 tablespoons of peanut butter, a cup of fat-free milk, decaffeinated coffee, and an orange.

Lunch

For lunch, you can have a spinach salad comprising of fresh spinach leaves, a sliced pear, ½ cup of canned sections of mandarin orange, 1/3 cup of slivered almonds, and 2 tablespoons of vinaigrette. The salad should be accompanied with 12 wheat crackers with low sodium content and a cup of fat-free milk.

Dinner

For dinner, prepare a herb-crusted baked cod, with 3 ounces of it cooked. This should be accompanied by ½ a cup of rice pilaf and an equal amount of steamed green beans, a small sourdough roll, a cup of fresh berries, and herbal iced tea.

Snack

Fat-free yogurt and 4 vanilla wafers can be taken as snacks in between meals.

Day 2

Breakfast

1 bran muffin to accompany a cup of herbal tea is enough for breakfast. You can add a fruit salad.

Lunch

Prepare curried chicken wrap for lunch. This is prepared using 1 medium sided whole-wheat tortilla, 2/3 cup of chopped chicken, cooked, ½ cup of chopped apple, 1 ½ tablespoon of mayonnaise and ½ teaspoons of curry powder. Accompanying it are a cup of raw baby carrots and a cup of fat-free milk.

Dinner

Have whole-wheat spaghetti with some side salad. Complete the meal with some sparkling clean water.

Snacks

For snacks, you can mix up a ¼ cup of raisins, an ounce of twist pretzels, and 2 tablespoons of sunflower seeds.

Day 3

Breakfast

A slice of whole-wheat toast, a banana, and a cup of fat-free milk are enough to act as your breakfast.

Lunch

Have Tuna salad made with a ¼ cup of diced celery, ½ cup of unsalted water-packed tuna, 2 tablespoons of light mayonnaise, and 15 grapes. Accompanying this is a cup of fat-free milk and 8 Melba toast crackers.

Dinner

Prepare a beef and vegetable kebab for dinner. The same should be accompanied by a cup of cooked rice, a cup of pineapple chunks, and Cran-raspberry spritzer.

Snack

1 medium peach and a cup of light yogurt can be snacked at any time.

Day 4

Breakfast

To start your day 4 of week three, a slice of whole wheat bread, one tablespoon of margarine, and a cup of fruit yogurt will do.

Lunch

For lunch, prepare a ham and cheese sandwich. You will need 2 whole-wheat bread slices, 2 ounces of ham, a slice of cheese, leafy lettuce, a tablespoon of mayonnaise, and 2 slices of tomatoes to prepare the meal.

Dinner

Prepare chicken with spinach rice. Serve with a cup of green peas and a cup of low-fat milk.

Snacks

¼ cup of apricots, a cup of apple juice, and 1/3 cup of almonds can be taken as snacks.

Day 5

Breakfast

A banana, a cup of low-fat milk, medium raisin bagel, a tablespoon of peanut butter, and a cup of orange juice should be enough to get you started on your day.

Lunch

Prepare a tuna salad plate for lunch. Accompany it with cucumber salad and some fresh fruit juice.

Dinner

Prepare a 3-ounce turkey meatloaf together with some baked potatoes and a cup of collard greens for dinner.

Snacks

A cup of fruit yogurt and 2 tablespoons of sunflower seeds can be taken as snacks.

Day 6

Breakfast

For breakfast, 1 bar of granola, a banana, ½ a cup of fat-free fruit yogurt, and a cup of orange juice are great for breakfast.

Lunch

For lunch, a turkey breast sandwich made with 3 ounces of turkey breast, 2 slices of whole-wheat bread, 2 tablespoons of mayonnaise, and a tablespoon of Dijon mustard is a good choice.

Dinner

Prepare 3 ounces of spicy baked fish served with a cup of scallion rice, ½ cup of spinach, and a cup of cooked carrots.

Snacks

For snacking in between meals, take 2 tablespoons of peanut butter, ¼ cup of apricots, and a cup of low-fat milk.

Day 7

Breakfast

For breakfast, you will need a cup of whole-grain oat rings, a banana, and a cup of low-fat milk. A cup of fruit yogurt completes the meal.

Lunch

For lunch, you can have a tuna salad sandwich, an apple and a cup of low-fat milk.

Dinner

To complete the week, you will need a cup of fresh spinach, 2 tablespoons of croutons, a tablespoon of vinaigrette, a tablespoon of sunflower seed, a whole-wheat roll, and a cup of grape juice.

Snacks

For snacks in between meals, 1/3 cup of unsalted almonds, ¼ cup of apricots, and 6 whole-wheat crackers will serve the purpose.

Week 4

Day 1

Breakfast

1 cup of skim milk, a cup of oatmeal, ½ cup of blueberries, and a cup of fresh orange juice to start off your day.

Lunch

For lunch, prepare a tuna and mayonnaise sandwich. Use 2 slices of whole-wheat bread, a tablespoon of mayonnaise, 1 ½ cup of green salad, and 3 ounces of canned tuna.

Dinner

Your dinner can be made of 3 ounces of lean chicken breast. It should be cooked in 1 teaspoon of vegetable oil and accompanied with a cup of brown rice served with ½ cup each of carrots and broccoli.

Snacks

1 medium apple or a banana can be snacked in between meals.

Day 2

Breakfast

On the second day of week 4, take 2 slices of whole-grain toast with a tablespoon of jam or jelly and ½ a cup of fresh orange juice for breakfast. Finish with an apple.

Lunch

For lunch, prepare lean chicken breasts, 3 ounces, with 2 cups of green salad. The same should be accompanied by a cup of brown rice and 1.5 ounces of cheese.

Dinner

Prepare 3 ounces of salmon. It should be prepared in a tablespoon of vegetable oil and served with 1.5 cups of boiled veggies and a cup of boiled potatoes.

Snack

A banana or 1 cup of low-fat yogurt and ½ a cup of canned peaches can be snacked in between meals.

Day 3

Breakfast

On day 3, start your day with a cup of oatmeal, a cup of skim milk, ½ a cup of fresh orange juice, and an equal amount of blueberries.

Lunch

For lunch, prepare a sandwich made with 2 slices of white-grain bread, 3 ounces of lean turkey, and 1.5 ounces of low-fat cheese. Also, add ½ a cup of green salad and an equal amount of cherry tomatoes.

Dinner

Dinner on day 3 is made up of 6 ounces of cod fillet, a cup of mashed potatoes, ½ a cup of broccoli, and an equal amount of green peas.

Snack

4 whole-wheat crackers together with ½ a cup of canned pineapple are great for snacks.

Day 4

Breakfast

1 cup of skim milk with a cup of oatmeal and ½ cup of raspberries. Add ½ cup of fresh orange juice to complete your breakfast meal.

Lunch

Prepare a salad for lunch. The salad is made of 4.5 ounces of grilled tuna, 2 cups of greens, one boiled egg, and ½ a cup of cherry tomatoes.

Dinner

For dinner, prepare pork fillet, 3 ounces, together with a cup of brown rice, and an equal amount of mixed vegetables.

Snacks

A cup of low-fat yogurt accompanying ½ a cup of canned pears can be used as snacks between the meals. A banana can work too.

Day 5

Breakfast

For breakfast, have 2 boiled eggs, ½ a cup of baked beans, 2 turkey bacon slices with ½ a cup of cherry tomatoes plus a ½ cup of fresh orange juice.

Lunch

2 whole-wheat toast slices, 1.5 low-fat cheese ounces, ½ cup of greens, and ½ a cup of cherry tomatoes for lunch will do fine.

Dinner

For dinner, prepare meatballs and spaghetti, with ½ a cup of green peas.

Snack

An apple or fruit salad to be snacked

Day 6

Breakfast

On day 6 of week 4, breakfast should comprise of 2 whole-wheat toast slices with 2 tablespoons of peanut butter, a banana, and ½ a cup of orange juice.

Lunch

3 ounces of grilled chicken and a cup of low-fat yogurt will do it for lunch.

Dinner

Prepare 3 ounces of pork steak with a cup of brown rice. Serve it with ½ cup of lentils. Also, add 1.5 ounces of low-fat cheese into the mix. A chocolate pudding can be taken as dessert.

Snack

An apple or a cup of low-fat yogurt.

Day 7

Breakfast

For day 28 of the meal plan, take a cup of oatmeal together with a cup of skim milk, half a cup of blueberries, and an equal amount of fresh orange juice for breakfast.

Lunch

Chicken salad with 3 ounces of meat and 2 cups of greens, ½ a cup of cherry tomatoes, ½ a tablespoon of seeds, and 4 whole-wheat crackers for lunch.

Dinner

For dinner, prepare 3 ounces of roast beef, alongside a cup of boiled potatoes, ½ a cup of green peas, and ½ a cup of broccoli.

Snacks

A pear, a banana, or ½ a cup of almonds are great for snacks.

Shopping for ingredients for the meal plan

This meal plan comprises of so many ingredients. It can be quite overwhelming to do a one-time shopping for all 28 days. To make it easier and to ensure you do not miss anything you need during the period, do your grocery shopping on a weekly basis. At the end of every week, list down all the ingredients you will need to have when preparing your meals the following week and shop for them. This will ensure that you have everything you need. Also, this method ensures that you get fresh products.

Chapter 8: The Recipes, Meal Plans, Ingredient, and the Cooking Instructions That You Should Follow

Week 1

Day 1

Breakfast

Cooking time: 10-30 minutes

Ingredients

- Hard-boiled eggs
- Bacon slice
- 6 ounces of low sodium tomato juice

Cooking instructions

1. Heat water until it becomes hot, pick 4 eggs and boil them to hard level.
2. Fry the bacon till golden brown on both sides.
3. Serve while hot with tomato juice

Midmorning snack

Preparation time: 5 minutes

- Baby carrots and a stick light cheese

Lunch

Cooking time: 10-30 mins

Ingredients

- Quinoa meatless balls and cherry tomatoes
- A side salad with vinegar dressing and a cup of Strawberry Jell-O

Cooking instructions

1. Heat the vegetable oil in a separate bowl. Form meatballs and cook over for 3 minutes.
2. Prepare the sauce in a bowl, heat olive oil and add ingredients and cook for 10 minutes.
3. Add lime juice, coconut milk, and vegetable broth and let it heat for 7 minutes.
4. Add chopped cilantro and set aside.
5. Place the meatballs in the sauce for 10 minutes.
6. Serve quinoa with the side salad with vinegar dressing and a cup of Strawberry Jell-O

Afternoon Snack

A handful of cashews and 4 ounces of lemon light yogurt

Dinner

Ingredients

- Chicken Kabobs with salad
- A cup of sugar-free raspberry Jell-O

Cooking time: 10-30 mins

Cooking instructions

1. Heat coals.
2. Cover and grill kabob 6 inches from medium heat, 20 minutes
3. Serve with reserved 1/2 cup dressing.
4. Stir in 2 cups of water then cool for 4 hours. Add 1 cups of boiling water to the mix and stir.
5. Serve them together when hot.

Day 2

Breakfast

Ingredients

- A fried omelet
- 4-5 ounces of low-sodium tomato juice

Cooking time: 5 minutes

Cooking instructions

1. Beat eggs and the ingredients in small bowl until blended.
2. Heat butter in omelet pan until hot. Pour in egg mixture.
3. Continue cooking while tilting pan
4. Serve immediately with the tomato juice.

Midmorning snack

- A cheese wedge slice
- 6 grape tomatoes

Lunch

Ingredients

- Have 2 Turkey-Swiss roll-ups with cheese wrappings on the outside
- A cup of coleslaw and a cup of sugar-free Orange Jell-O

Cooking time: 10-30 mins

Cooking instructions

1. Spread a teaspoon of mayonnaise on the inside of outer leaf of iceberg.
2. Place a leaf on the table and top with the slices
3. Add some cheese on the outside
4. Serve with a cup of coleslaw when done

Afternoon Snack

10 peanuts will be enough to keep you going until dinner time.

Dinner

Ingredients

- Roasted sliced turkey served with sautéed onions and carrot.
- A side salad and a cup of sugar-free Lime Jell-O.

Cooking time 10-30 mins

Cooking instructions

- Heat oven.
- Remove the turkey neck and rinse it.
- Fill the body with stuffing, salt, and pepper.
- Place turkey in the oven. Roast for 5 hours.

- Add a salad to the side when done.
- Serve with lime Jell-O.

Day 3

Breakfast

Ingredients

- Scrambled eggs
- A slice or two of Canadian bacon
- 4 ounces of cranberry juice

Cooking time 5 minutes

Cooking instructions

1. Beat eggs and the ingredients of milk, salt, and pepper in a bowl.
2. Heat butter in a big pan until hot then you can add egg mixture.
3. Pull the eggs across the pan.
4. Fry the bacon till golden brown on both sides.
5. Serve with cranberry juice when hot.

Midmorning Snack

Your mid-morning snack could be made of 4 ounces of light low-fat yogurt and ¼ cup of almonds.

Lunch

Ingredients

- Fried chicken breasts with no skin
- Coleslaw
- Baby carrots will do for lunch
- A cup of lemon Jell-O

Cooking time: 10 mins

Cooking instructions

1. Cut the whole chickens
2. Heat your oil. In a large bowl, combine the ingredients.
3. Pour the buttermilk into another bowl.
4. Place your chicken in a bowl with buttermilk and then next in dry mixture.
5. Place the breasts in your hot oil for cooking for 15 minutes.
6. Add coleslaw and baby carrots on top.
7. Serve with lemon jell when hot.

Afternoon Snack

6 grape tomatoes and a slice cheese wedges

Dinner

Ingredients

- Turkey burger

- A cup of broccoli and
- A side salad
- A cup or two of sugar-free strawberry Jell-O.

Cooking time: 10 mins

Cooking instructions

1. Peel the onions in the same bowl, add the wheat germ, salt, turkey, barbecue sauce, oats, and pepper
2. Cook the burgers while flipping until golden brown.
3. Add a cup of broccoli and side salad to it.
4. Serve with strawberry jell while hot.

Day 4

Breakfast

Ingredients

- 8 ounces of skim milk
- ¾ cup of Wheaties
- 4-6 ounces of raspberries or strawberries.

Cooking time: 10 mins

Preparation

- Mix the Wheaties and skim milk
- Add some raspberries and strawberries

Midmorning Snack

The optional midmorning snack could be made of a light cheese wedge and grape tomatoes.

Lunch

Ingredients

- 2-3 Swiss and turkey roll-ups
- Baby carrots and small plum

Cooking time: 10 mins

Cooking instructions

1. Lay your tortillas on a flat table and put avocado onto each tortilla.
2. Then the turkey, spinach, Swiss cheese, and bacon over 4 of the tortilla.
3. Roll the tortilla tightly.
4. Slice into pinwheels and serve.
5. Add baby carrots and small plum and serve them together

Afternoon Snack

10 cashews and 6 ounces of blueberry yogurt should be more than enough for you.

Dinner

Ingredients

- Tilapia
- Olive oil
- Butter
- Melon salsa

Cooking instructions

1. Heat olive oil and cook the tilapia at least 5 minutes while flipping.
2. Accompany the fish with mango-melon salsa and a cup of strawberry Jell-O.
3. Serve and enjoy.

Day 5

Breakfast

Ingredients

- Hot chocolate
- 2 hard-boiled eggs
- Light cranberry juice

Cooking time: 5 mins

Cooking instructions

1. Put eggs in a pan and cover with hot water for 15 minutes
2. Drain eggs lastly then put in a cold bowl of water
3. Serve and enjoy

Midmorning Snack

10 ounces of almonds together with 6 ounces of lime yogurt will do just fine.

Lunch

Ingredients

Swiss and Turkey Sandwich

Cooking instructions

1. Put 3 ounces of turkey and a slice of Swiss cheese on two whole wheat bread slices

2. Add the ingredients

3. Accompany with Raspberry Jell-O cup

Afternoon Snack

Pepper strips and a half a cup of hummus.

Dinner

Ingredients

- Vegetable and Quinoa.
- Fudge bar and a side salad with vinaigrette or Italian dressing.

Cooking time: 20 minutes

Cooking instructions

1. Fry the vegetable and stir them together with quinoa

2. Add fudge and a slide salad

3. Serve them while hot

Day 6

Breakfast

Ingredients

- ½ cup oatmeal
- Half a banana
- 6 ounces of tomato juice and latte

Cooking time: 5 mins

Cooking instructions

1. Cookout the meal with the right amount of heat
2. Add banana to the menu and serve with tomato juice and latte

Midmorning Snack

Baby carrot and a stick light cheese are good for a midmorning snack.

Lunch

Ingredients

- Three-Bean kale
- Brown rice served with sliced bell peppers
- Orange Jell-O cup.

Cooking time: 15 mins

Cooking instructions

1. Heat olive oil and add onion and garlic slices together
2. Cover them with a lead and let it cook for 13 minutes
3. Serve when hot

Afternoon Snack

For snacks, you can have 10 cashews and 4-6 ounces of strawberries.

Dinner

Ingredients

- White bean
- Cabbage soup
- Green beans
- Side salad
- Frozen yogurt

Cooking time: 20 minutes

Cooking instructions

1. Prepare cabbage soup with white bean together for 10 minutes
2. Prepare tomatoes with a side and salad green beans
3. Serve them together with frozen yogurt when hot

Day 7

Breakfast

Ingredients

- 1-3 scrambled eggs
- A slice of a light whole-wheat toast
- Tablespoon of jam or jelly
- 4 ounces of orange juice and 8 ounces of skim milk or latte.

Cooking time: 10 minutes

Cooking instructions

1. Beat eggs and the other ingredients together in a bowl.
2. Heat butter in pan until hot then pour in egg mixture.
3. Continue cooking until no liquid remains on the egg.
4. Serve while hot.

Midmorning Snack

4-6 ounces blueberries together with 10 almonds should be enough for a midmorning snack.

Lunch

Ingredients

- 3 roast beef
- Muenster cheese

- Italian coleslaw
- Small peach

Cooking instructions

1. Muenster cheese and 2 roast beef roll-ups together with Italian coleslaw.
2. Prepare some Italian coleslaw grated carrots with oil.
3. Serve and enjoy

Afternoon Snack

6 ounces of artificially sweetened strawberry light yogurt.

Dinner

Ingredients

- Salmon stuffed avocado
- A side salad and a low-fat bar of ice cream.

Cooking time: 10mins

Cooking instructions

1. Place scooped avocado into an average bowl. Mix with a fork.
2. Add Salmon. Pour lime juice over and stir then add bell pepper and cilantro to the bowl.
3. Add a side salad and a low-fat bar of ice cream and serve them together

Week 2

Day 1

Breakfast

Ingredients

- Egg toast
- Salsa wheat bread
- Pepper
- salt

Preparation time: 5 mins

Cooking instructions

1. Prepare egg toast with frying pan using pepper and salt
2. Serve with wheat bread while hot

Midmorning Snack

Cinnamon pears will serve you well as a midmorning snack. Slice the pear and sprinkle cinnamon over the slices.

Lunch

Ingredients

- Veggie-hummus sandwich
- Simple snack calories

Cooking instructions

1. Prepare a veggie-hummus sandwich for lunch.
2. Serve with a simple snack carries 325 calories.

Afternoon Snack

For your afternoon snack, you can have ¾ cup of raspberries and any fruit juice.

Dinner

Ingredients

- Lemmon-herb salmon
- Caponata
- Farro
- Side salad
- Yogurt

Cooking time: 15 mins

Cooking instructions

1. Caponata and Farro served with Lemmon-Herb salmon
2. A side salad and light and accompany with yogurt.

Day 2

Breakfast

Ingredients

- Fig and honey yogurt
- 2/3 cup nonfat
- plain yogurt
- 5 dried and chopped figs
- 2 teaspoons of chia seeds
- 1 and ½ teaspoons of honey

Cooking instructions

The yogurt is prepared by simply topping the plain yogurt with the figs, honey, and chia seeds.

Midmorning Snack

Have yourself ½ a cup of grapes for a midmorning snack.

Lunch

Ingredients

- White bean together with avocado salad
- Mixed greens
- ¾ cup of chopped vegetables
- 1/3 cup of canned white beans
- ½ avocado that has been diced
- 2 tablespoons of all-purpose vinaigrette

- Top salad greens with the beans, avocado, veggies, and vinaigrette.

Cooking time: 20 mins

Cooking instructions

1. Whisk together the olive oil in a bowl. Add salt, pepper, lemon juice
2. In another bowl, mix together the basil, avocado, beans, and tomatoes
3. Coat the salad. Serve while hot and enjoy

Afternoon Snack

Have yourself 1 clementine for the afternoon.

Dinner

Ingredients

- Cauliflower steaks
- Tzatziki
- Red rice
- Nut butter bites

Cooking instructions

1. Prepare cauliflower steaks with Tzatziki and Red rice.
2. Serve with nut and chocolate butter

Day 3

Breakfast

Ingredients

- Cinnamon toast
- Latte

Cooking time: 7 minutes

Cooking instructions

1. Butter a slice of bread.
2. Place cinnamon in a bowl then stir them with sugar to combine.
3. Sprinkle the cinnamon on top of the butter for 8 minutes.
4. Serve and enjoy

Midmorning Snack

A cup of raspberries should complete your morning meal perfectly.

Lunch

Ingredients

- Beef sandwich
- Veggies
- Cheese slice wheat bread
- Grapes

Cooking time: 10 minutes

Cooking instructions

1. Place a slice of well-fried beef, veggies, and a slice of cheese
2. Accompany with a cup of grapes.

Afternoon snack

Ingredients

Pears

Preparation time: 5 mins

Preparation method

- Slice the pear into pieces and sprinkle cinnamon on the pieces.
- Serve and enjoy

Dinner

Ingredients

- Mediterranean chicken
- Orzo salad
- 1 clementine
- 2 chicken breast
- Olive oil

- Lemmon zest
- ½ teaspoon of salt
- ½ teaspoon of ground pepper
- ¾ cup of whole-wheat orzo
- 2 cups of sliced baby spinach
- A cup of chopped cucumber
- A cup of chopped tomato
- ¼ cups of red onion, chopped, ¼ cup of crumbled feta cheese
- 2 tablespoons of Kalamata olives, chopped
- 2 tablespoons of lemon juice
- 1 clove of grated garlic

Cooking instructions

1. Anoint the chicken with oil and salt then bake for 25 minutes
2. Add water in a pan and boil together with orzo and let it cook for 5 minutes
3. Cook for a minute then drain. Add the ingredients then stir
4. Serve and enjoy

Day 4

Breakfast

Ingredient

- Yogurt and raspberries
- Cup of plain yogurt
- ½ a cup of raspberries
- 5 chopped walnuts and 1 tablespoon of honey

Cooking instruction

1. Simply top the yogurt with the other ingredients.
2. Serve and enjoy

Midmorning Snack

Slices of a whole apple with cinnamon sprinkled on them is enough.

Lunch

Ingredients

- White bean with avocado toast
- A side salad of salad greens topped with carrots
- Cucumber and vinaigrette

Cooking instructions

1. Place the bread in the toaster and toast it
2. Go on to place Colavita Olive Oil as an addition

3. Add salt and pepper for seasoning
4. Take the avocado mash and spread it on the toast
5. Scoop a spoon of white beans and place it on top of each piece
6. Take hot pepper and sprinkle as well as parsley
7. Add side salad together with carrots and accompany with cucumber
8. Serve and enjoy

Afternoon Snack

1 medium plum

Dinner

Ingredients

1. Sweet potatoes dressed with a hummus dressing
2. 1 cup of chopped kale
3. A cup of canned black beans
4. 1 cup of hummus and 2 tablespoons of water

Cooking time: 15 minutes

Cooking instructions

1. Prick the sweet potato and put it in a microwave for 10 minutes
2. Place kales in a pan, cover and let it cook for 10 minutes with less water

3. Drizzle the dressing over the sweet potato
4. Serve while hot

Day 5

Breakfast

Ingredients

Prepare a peanut-butter cinnamon toast.

Cooking time: 10 minutes

Cooking instructions

1. Heat oven, combine the sugar and cinnamon
2. Put the bread on a baking sheet and bake for 9 minutes
3. Spread bread with peanut butter. Make a sandwich and cut in half. Serve immediately.

Midmorning Snack

2 clementine is enough to wrap up the morning meals

Lunch

Ingredients

A green salad with some pita bread and hummus

Cooking instructions

1. Top greens with cucumber, vinaigrette, and carrot.
2. Serve with the pita bread and hummus.
3. Serve with medium plum.

Afternoon Snack

A cup of grapes

Dinner

Ingredients

- Chicken chili with sweet potatoes, coupled
- ¼ diced avocado and 1 tablespoon of nonfat plain yogurt

Cooking instructions

1. Heat oil then add the ingredients that are available
2. Add the chicken pieces to it then fry it for 4 minutes
3. Heat vegetable oil then add spring onions and fry
4. Add the ingredients and stir
5. Add the fried chicken pieces and stir well Serve warm with some noodles and yogurt

Day 6

Breakfast

Ingredients

Start your day 6 with a fig and honey yogurt for breakfast.

Preparation: 5 minutes

Preparation method

It is prepared by topping plain Greek yogurt with dried figs, 2 tablespoons of chia seed, and 1 ½ teaspoon of honey.

Midmorning Snack

A cup of raspberries will do just fine for your midmorning snack.

Lunch

Ingredients

- Turkey with Pear Pita Melt
- ½ whole-wheat pita round
- Large, 3 ½ oz. deli turkey with low sodium levels
- 1 sliced medium-sized pear
- A tablespoon of shredded cheddar cheese and a cup of mixed greens

Cooking instructions

1. Use the turkey and cheese. Toast in an oven and add green onto the pita when serving. The remaining pear slices should be served on the side.

Afternoon Snack

1 medium plum

Dinner

Ingredients

- A lemon-garlic shrimp served over orzo and zucchini
- One clementine and a serving of nut and chocolate bites.

Cooking time: 40 minutes

Cooking instructions

1. Cook orzo and drain
2. Heat the butter then add shrimp and cook 7 minutes
3. Heat the remaining then add ingredients then cook for 10 minutes
4. Stir orzo mixture into shrimp mixture and sprinkle with dill and lemon slivers
5. Serve

Day 7

Breakfast

Ingredients

- An egg toast with salsa.
- A slice of whole-wheat bread with egg
- Pepper, salt, and salsa

Cooking time: 10 minutes

Cooking instructions

1. Spread avocado mash onto toast
2. Warm olive oil and place an egg into the heated pan and cook
3. Top avocado with egg and salsa
4. Toast a slice of whole wheat with eggs, serve and enjoy

Midmorning Snack

A banana

Lunch

Ingredients

- Chicken Chili
- Sweet potatoes

Cooking time: 25 minutes

Cooking instructions

1. Heat oil and add onion, sweet potato, and salt; cook for 5 minutes
2. Add beans and boil for 10 minutes
3. Increase heat and stir for 3 minutes. Add chicken
4. Serve topped with sour cream

Afternoon Snack

½ cup of raspberries

Dinner

Ingredients

Chicken kabobs with salad and a cup of sugar-free raspberry Jell-O.

Cooking time: 30 minutes

Cooking instructions

1. Marinate the chicken overnight.
2. Soak in water at least 20 minutes if grilling outdoors.
3. Combine the first 10 salad ingredients and lay aside in cool freezer
4. Place the chicken on 3 skewers and cook on a hot grill for about 10 minutes.
5. Divide lettuce between 5 plates, top with salad
6. Serve with lemon wedges.

Week 3

Day 1

Breakfast

Ingredients

- 1 bagel or whole wheat with 2 tablespoons of peanut butter
- A cup of fat-free milk, decaffeinated coffee, and an orange

Preparation time: 5 minutes

Preparation instructions

Toast bagel. Spread peanut butter on bagel halves. Serve with orange.

Lunch

Ingredients

Spinach leaves, a sliced pear, ½ cup of canned sections of mandarin orange, a third (1/3) cup of slivered almonds, and 2 tablespoons of vinaigrette. The salad should be accompanied with 12 wheat crackers with low sodium content and a cup of fat-free milk.

Cooking instructions

1. Apply heat, grease and pour flour on the muffin pans
2. Mix flour and the other ingredients plus eggs
3. Pour sour cream into the mixture of the flour and stir it until it is moistened
4. Bake for 30 or 20 minutes up to when you will notice that the top is a bit brown
5. Serve with side salad and enjoy

Dinner

Ingredients

Herb-crusted baked cod, with 3 ounces of it cooked. This should be accompanied by ½ a cup of rice pilaf, and an equal amount of steamed green beans, a small sourdough roll, a cup of fresh berries and herbal iced tea.

Cooking time: 30 minutes

Cooking instructions

1. Heat the oven and lightly brush a baking sheet with olive oil
2. Anoint tomatoes with olive oil, salt. Roast 8 minutes
3. Place tomatoes and garlic to a blender when done. Add vinegar and 2 tablespoons of water
4. Chop the garlic clove. Add the ingredients. Add the bread crumbs, stirring with salt

5. Brush the cod fillets with olive oil and then dredge in the herb and bread crumb mixture, cook for 10 minutes

6. Serve the roasted cod on the sauce

Snack

Fat-free yogurt and 4 vanilla wafers can be taken as snacks in between meals.

Day 2

Breakfast

Ingredients

- 1 bran muffin to accompany a cup of herbal tea
- Fruit salad

Preparation time: 20 minutes

Preparation method

1. Heat oven. Grease muffin cups
2. Mix together wheat bran and buttermilk; let it stand for 8 minutes.
3. Beat together oil, egg, sugar, and vanilla and add to buttermilk/bran mixture and other ingredients then bake for 16 minutes.
4. Accompany with tea and enjoy.

Lunch

Ingredients

Prepare curried chicken wrap for lunch

Cooking time: 20 minutes

Cooking instructions

This is prepared using 1 medium sided whole-wheat tortilla, 2/3 cup of chopped chicken, cooked, ½ cup of chopped apple, 1

½ tablespoon of mayonnaise and ½ teaspoons of curry powder. Accompanying it are a cup of raw baby carrots and a cup of fat-free milk.

Dinner

Ingredients

Have whole-wheat spaghetti with some side salad

Cooking time: 10 minutes

Cooking instructions

1. Boil hot water and add spaghetti
2. Stir with pepper and salt till 5 minutes
3. Complete the meal with some sparkling clean water

Snacks

For snacks, you can mix up a ¼ cup of raisins, an ounce of twist pretzels, and 2 tablespoons of sunflower seeds.

Day 3

Breakfast

Ingredients

- A slice of whole-wheat toast
- A banana and a cup of fat-free milk

Preparation time: 5 minutes

Preparation method

1. Smear butter on the whole-wheat toast
2. Add some banana to the menu and a cup of fat-free milk
3. Serve and enjoy

Lunch

Ingredients

- Tuna salad made with a ¼ cup of diced celery
- ½ cup of unsalted water-packed tuna
- 2 tablespoons of light mayonnaise and 15 grapes
- Accompanying this is a cup of fat-free milk and 8 Melba toast crackers

Cooking time: 15 minutes

Cooking instructions

1. In a bowl, combine tuna, Greek yogurt, celery, onion, lemon juice, and garlic powder.

2. Place eggs in a saucepan and cover with cold water. Bring to a boil. Cover eggs with a tight-fitting lid for 8-10 minutes. Drain.

3. Place lettuce leaves into meal prep containers. Top with tuna mixture, eggs, almonds, cucumber, and apple.

4. Serve

Dinner

Ingredients

- Beef and vegetable kebab
- The same should be accompanied by a cup of cooked rice, a cup of pineapple chunks, and Crank's raspberry spritzer.

Cooking time: 20 minutes

Cooking instructions

1. Prepare beef and vegetable oil and fry
2. Accompany with a cup of cooked rice
3. A cup of pineapple chunks and raspberry accompanied during serving

Snack

1 medium peach and a cup of light yogurt can be snacked at any time

Day 4

Breakfast

Ingredients

- A slice of whole wheat bread
- One tablespoon of margarine and a cup of fruit yogurt

Preparation: 5 minutes

Preparation method

Smear butter to wheat bread and accompany it with fruit yogurt

Lunch

Ingredients

- Ham and cheese sandwich
- 2 whole-wheat bread slices
- 2 ounces of ham
- A slice of cheese
- Leafy lettuce
- A tablespoon of mayonnaise and 2 slices of tomatoes to prepare the meal

Cooking time: 5 minutes

Cooking instructions

1. Spread one side of each slice of bread with 1 teaspoon butter

2. Top with Swiss cheese and ham
3. Cook until the sandwich is golden brown and the cheese is melted about 6 minutes.
4. Serve

Dinner

Ingredients

- Prepare chicken with spinach rice
- Serve with a cup of green peas and a cup of low-fat milk

Cooking time: 30 minutes

Cooking instruction

1. Toss the chicken breast with salt
2. Heat olive oil then add chicken breast and cook until brown
3. Stir in rice and chicken. Boil and cover. Cook for 20 minutes
4. Remove pan from heat and place spinach on the rice. Let sit for 5 minutes.
5. Remove lid and stir well. Stir in cream and serve.

Snacks

¼ cup of apricots, a cup of apple juice and 1/3 cup of almonds can be taken as snacks.

Day 5

Breakfast

Ingredients

- A banana
- A cup of low-fat milk
- Medium raisin bagel
- A tablespoon of peanut butter and a cup of orange juice

Preparation time: 5 minutes

Preparation method

1. Add an egg and honey to the mixture for a sweet, crispy bagel
2. Add a dash of pepper
3. Serve accompanied with banana and orange juice

Lunch

Ingredients

- Tuna salad plate
- Cucumber salad and some fresh fruit juice

Cooking time: 1 hour

Cooking instructions

1. Drain tuna
2. Add the tuna to a bowl

3. Stir in the rest of your ingredients
4. Mix well and season to taste with salt and pepper. Let it for 1 hour
5. Serve with fresh juice and enjoy

Dinner

Ingredients

- 3-ounce turkey meatloaf
- Baked potatoes
- A cup of collard greens for dinner

Cooking time: 1 hour

Cooking instructions

1. In a bowl, combine 3 tbsp. ketchup with Worcestershire sauce.
2. Boil olive oil and onion on low until translucent, remove from heat.
3. In a bowl mix turkey, onion, egg, ½ cup ketchup, and salt.
4. Place mixture into a loaf pan and place on a baking pan.
5. Bake uncovered for 50 minutes. Remove from oven and let it sit for 10 minutes.
6. Serve

Snacks

A cup of fruit yogurt and 2 tablespoons of sunflower seeds can be taken as snacks.

Day 6

Breakfast

Ingredients

- 1 bar of granola
- A banana
- ½ a cup of fat-free fruit yogurt and a cup of orange juice are great for breakfast

Preparation time: 5 minutes

Preparation method

Eat granola accompanied with fruit, yogurt, and banana

Lunch

Ingredients

- Turkey breast sandwich made with 3 ounces of turkey breast
- 2 slices of whole-wheat bread
- 2 tablespoons of mayonnaise and a tablespoon of Dijon mustard

Cooking time: 30 minutes

Cooking instructions

1. Place the herbs and butter into the bowl of a food processor and pulse until green

2. Add avocado slices, crispy bacon slices, lettuce, and another slice of fontina cheese

3. Serve

Dinner

Ingredients

- Prepare 3 ounces of spicy baked fish served with a cup of scallion rice

- ½ cup of spinach and a cup of cooked carrots.

Cooking time: 40 minutes

Cooking instructions

1. Heat oven. Place cod fillets in baking pan. Bake for 20 minutes.

2. Heat a little oil in a saucepan and then cook for 10 minutes with all the ingredients

3. Pour sauce over fish, sprinkle with sesame seeds and return to the oven for 13 minutes.

4. Sprinkle with chopped coriander.

5. Serve accompanied with scallion rice and cup of spinach.

Snacks

Take 2 tablespoons of peanut butter, ¼ cup of apricots and a cup of low-fat milk.

Day 7

Breakfast

Ingredients

- A cup of whole-grain oat rings, a banana, and a cup of low-fat milk
- A cup of fruit yogurt completes the meal

Preparation time: 5 minutes

Preparation method

Prepare whole grains oat rings and accompany it with banana and low-fat milk

Lunch

Ingredients

Tuna salad sandwich, an apple, and a cup of low-fat milk

Cooking time: 1 hour

Cooking instructions

1. In a medium bowl, mix the tuna, celery, onion, mayonnaise, lemon juice, salt, and pepper.
2. Spread tuna mixture on 4 bread slices. Top with remaining bread slices.

Dinner

Ingredients

a cup of fresh spinach, 2 tablespoons of croutons, a tablespoon of vinaigrette, a tablespoon of sunflower seed, a whole-wheat roll, and a cup of grape juice

Cooking time: 15 minutes

Cooking instructions

1. Heat 3 tbsp. olive oil in a bowl. Add the garlic and sauté for about 1 minute.
2. Add spinach to the pan
3. Remove from pan and drain excess liquid
4. Serve with grape juice

Snacks

For snacks in between meals, 1/3 cup of unsalted almonds, ¼ cup of apricots and 6 whole-wheat crackers will serve the purpose.

Week 4

Day 1

Breakfast

Ingredients

1 cup of skim milk, a cup of oatmeal, ½ cup of blueberries, and a cup of fresh orange juice to start off your day

Preparation time: 5 minutes

Preparation method

- Pour skim milk to oatmeal and blueberries on top
- Serve with orange juice

Lunch

Ingredients

- Tuna and mayonnaise sandwich
- Use 2 slices of whole-wheat bread, a tablespoon of mayonnaise
- 1 ½ cup of green salad and 3 ounces of canned tuna

Cooking time: 1 hour

Cooking instructions

1. In a medium bowl, mix the tuna, celery, onion, mayonnaise, lemon juice, salt, and pepper.

2. Spread tuna mixture on 4 bread slices. Top with remaining bread slices.

Dinner

Ingredients

- 3 ounces of lean chicken breast
- 1 teaspoon of vegetable oil
- A cup of brown rice served with ½ cup each of carrots and broccoli

Cooking time: 40 minutes

Cooking instructions

1. 3 ounces of lean chicken breast. Cooked in 1 teaspoon of vegetable oil and accompanied with a cup of brown rice served with ½ cup each of carrots and broccoli.
2. Serve when hot.

Snacks

1 medium apple or a banana can be snacked in between meals.

Day 2

Breakfast

Ingredients

- 2 slices of whole-grain toast with a tablespoon of jam or jelly
- ½ a cup of fresh orange juice for breakfast
- An apple

Preparation time: 5 minutes

Preparation method

On the second day of week 4, take 2 slices of whole-grain toast with a tablespoon of jam or jelly and ½ a cup of fresh orange juice for breakfast. Finish with an apple.

Lunch

Ingredients

- Lean chicken breasts, 3 ounces, with 2 cups of green salad
- A cup of brown rice and 1.5 ounces of cheese

Cooking time: 40 minutes

Cooking instructions

1. Rinse and pat chicken breasts dry
2. Bake 30 minutes

3. Accompany with a cup of brown rice and cheese
4. Serve and enjoy

Dinner

Ingredients

Prepare 3 ounces of salmon. It should be prepared in a tablespoon of vegetable oil and served with 1.5 cups of boiled veggies and a cup of boiled potatoes.

Cooking time: 40 minutes

Cooking instructions

1. Melt the butter in a frying pan
2. Place the broccoli into a pan of boiling salted water and boil for 5 minutes
3. Pile the broccoli onto a serving plate and top with the pan-fried salmon
4. Serve with boiled veggies and boiled potatoes

Snack

A banana or 1 cup of low-fat yogurt and ½ a cup of canned peaches can be snacked in between meals.

Day 3

Breakfast

Ingredients

On day 3, start your day with a cup of oatmeal, a cup of skim milk, ½ a cup of fresh orange juice and an equal amount of blueberries.

Preparation time: 5 minutes

Preparation method

1. Mix oatmeal and skim milk together and blueberries at the top
2. Serve with fresh orange

Lunch

Ingredients

- A sandwich made with 2 slices of white-grain bread, 3 ounces of lean turkey
- 1.5 ounces of low-fat cheese
- Add ½ a cup of green salad and an equal amount of cherry tomatoes

Cooking time: 30 minutes

Cooking instructions

For lunch, prepare a sandwich made with 2 slices of white-grain bread, 3 ounces of lean turkey, and 1.5 ounces of low-fat cheese. Also, add ½ a cup of green salad and an equal amount of cherry tomatoes.

Dinner

Ingredients

Dinner on day 3 is made up of 6 ounces of cod fillet, a cup of mashed potatoes, ½ a cup of broccoli, and an equal amount of green peas.

Cooking time: 20 minutes

Cooking instructions

1. Spray a large rimmed baking sheet with non-stick spray.
2. Add the butter, lemon juice, parsley, salt, and pepper to a bowl and mix together.
3. Spread the butter mixture evenly over each cod filet and top with a slice of lemon.
4. Bake for 17 minutes.
5. Serve with broccoli and green peas.

Snack

4 whole-wheat crackers together with ½ a cup of canned pineapple is great for snacks.

Day 4

Breakfast

Ingredients

1 cup of skim milk with a cup of oatmeal and ½ cup of raspberries. Add ½ cup of fresh orange juice to complete your breakfast meal.

Preparation time: 5 minutes

Preparation method

1. Mix skim milk and oatmeal altogether with drops of raspberries
2. Serve with fresh orange

Lunch

Ingredients

- Prepare a salad for lunch. The salad is made of 4.5 ounces of grilled tuna, 2 cups of greens, one boiled egg, and ½ a cup of cherry tomatoes.

Cooking time: 5 minutes

Cooking instructions

1. Place salad greens in a salad bowl and top with ingredients. Pour dressing over salad.
2. Serve with grilled tuna and boiled egg.

Dinner

Ingredients

- For dinner, prepare pork fillet, 3 ounces, together with a cup of brown rice and an equal amount of mixed vegetables.

Cooking time: 20 minutes

Cooking instructions

1. Brush pork fillets with oil and sprinkle with pepper for 12 minutes.
2. Brush with combined vinegar, honey, oregano, and garlic.
3. Roast for 7 minutes and accompany with brown rice and vegetables. Serve when hot.

Snacks

A cup of low-fat yogurt accompanying ½ a cup of canned pears can be used as snacks between the meals. A banana too can work.

Day 5

Breakfast

Ingredients

For breakfast, have 2 boiled eggs, ½ a cup of baked beans, 2 turkey bacon slices with ½ a cup of cherry tomatoes plus a ½ cup of fresh orange juice.

Preparation time: 5 minutes

Preparation method

- Boil the eggs and prepare baked beans
- Fry turkey bacon till golden brown
- Serve with orange juice

Lunch

Ingredients

- 2 whole-wheat toast slices, 1.5 low-fat cheese ounces, ½ cup of greens, and ½ a cup of cherry tomatoes for lunch will do fine.

Cooking time: 7 minutes

Cooking instructions

1. Prepare low-fat cheese accompanied with greens and cherry tomatoes
2. Serve with two whole-wheat toast slices

3. Enjoy

Dinner

Ingredients

- For dinner, prepare meatballs and spaghetti, with ½ a cup of green peas.

Cooking time: 10 minutes

Cooking instructions

1. Prepare meatballs and store in a bog bowl
2. Boil hot water and add salt then pour spaghetti for 6 minutes while stirring
3. Serve with green peas
4. Serve while hot

Snack

An apple or fruit salad to be snacked.

Day 6

Breakfast

Ingredients

- 2 whole-wheat toast slices with 2 tablespoons of peanut butter
- A banana and ½ a cup of orange juice

Preparation time: 5 minutes

Preparation method

Smear peanut butter to the whole-white slices and serve with banana and orange juice

Lunch

Ingredients

3 ounces of grilled chicken and a cup of low-fat yogurt will do it for lunch

Cooking time: 40 minutes

Cooking instructions

1. In a bowl, mix garlic powder, sea salt, pepper, and olive oil and mix
2. Place chicken on grill and grill each side for 7 minutes
3. Serve with low-fat yogurt

Dinner

Ingredients

- 3 ounces of pork steak with a cup of brown rice
- ½ cup of lentils. Also, add 1.5 ounces of low-fat cheese into the mix
- A chocolate pudding can be taken as a dessert

Cooking time: 40 minutes

Cooking instruction

1. Melt butter in a pan and mix in the soy sauce
2. Place the pork steaks in the skillet, cover, and cook 9 minutes on each side
3. Serve with lentils and fat cheese together with chocolate pudding as dessert

Snack

An apple or a cup of low-fat yogurt

Day 7

Breakfast

Ingredients

- For day 28 of the meal plan, take a cup of oatmeal together with a cup of skim milk, half a cup of blueberries and an equal amount of fresh orange juice for breakfast.

Preparation time: 5 minutes

Preparation method

1. Mix oatmeal with skim milk and drops of blueberries
2. Serve with orange juice

Lunch

Ingredients

Chicken salad with 3 ounces of meat and 2 cups of greens, ½ a cup of cherry tomatoes, ½ a tablespoon of seeds, and 4 whole-wheat crackers for lunch

Cooking time: 40 minutes

Cooking instructions

1. Prep salad ingredient
2. Make the dressing
3. Taste for the proper balance of sweetness and acidity
4. Add more preserves
5. Add salt and pepper to taste
6. Serve with whole wheat crackers while hot

Dinner

Ingredients

For dinner, prepare 3 ounces of roast beef alongside a cup of boiled potatoes, ½ a cup of green peas, and ½ a cup of broccoli

Cooking time: 30 minutes

Cooking instructions

1. Place roast in pan and season with salt, garlic powder, and pepper. Add more or fewer seasonings to taste.
2. Roast in the oven
3. Serve with boiled potatoes and green peas with broccoli

Snacks

A pear, a banana or ½ a cup of almonds are great for snacks.

Summary

Ensure to go shopping every week so as not to miss out on anything and to have fresh groceries.

Conclusion

Congratulations to you for taking the time to learn how to implement the dash diet into your daily life and for doing it successfully! Thank you for reading the book and making it up to the end of it.

It is not easy to start upon something new, especially to change how you eat. However, if you have read this book, you are interested in making the change. Let this book be your first guide as a beginner starting on the diet. We hope that you have enjoyed reading the book and got as much information as possible. Before you embark on new diets, always make sure to consult your doctor.

If this book has helped you in any way, a review on Amazon will be appreciated!